Laughing in the Storm
Conquering Cancer with a Smile on Your Face

Jen Cerminara

First published by Dog Ear Publishing
4011 Vincennes Rd
Indianapolis, IN 46268
www.dogearpublishing.net

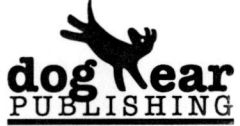

ISBN: 978-1-4575-5640-1

This book is printed on acid-free paper.

Printed in the United States of America

Front cover and About the Author photography by Kylie Randal

Acknowledgments

There are so many people I need to thank for helping me throughout this journey. My heart is full of love and gratitude, and I am truly blessed to have such amazing people in my life.

God: Without You, I wouldn't be here today. I can't even begin to thank You for what You have done for me, and what You continue to do for me every single day. Thank You for your grace, mercy, and this second chance at life.

Danielle, my sister, best friend, and fellow cancer warrior: What you have gone through and accomplished definitely inspired me to get through this crazy journey of mine. You have gone through so much but are now incredibly blessed with great health, a great job, and a bright future. You are proof that miracles exist. You inspire me every day. I love you.

Mom and Dad: I cannot thank you both enough for everything you have done for me, especially during the hardest year of my life. I love you both so very much. I appreciate everything more than you will ever know. I can't even imagine how hard it was for you to have two daughters battling cancer. Your strength and faith, however, kept me going. Your prayers and encouragement made me feel strong. Thank you, thank you, thank you.

Aunt Janis, another cancer warrior: You are incredibly tough and brave. I appreciate and love you very much. You really helped me during this difficult year, and my heart is overflowing with happiness because of our strong bond. Thank you for being not only my aunt but also one of my best friends.

Aunt Denise: Thank you for being such a huge part of my journey. I appreciate every single thing you have done for me more than you will ever know. It meant the world to me when you came wig shopping with me and bought me Sonia. I simply cannot thank you enough. I love you.

Grandma and Papa (two more cancer survivors) and Uncle John: You are all incredibly wonderful. Thank you for everything! Your love and support mean so much to me. I love you.

Blythe and Muriel, my two fellow warriors: I thank God every day that you are in my life, and that we were able to have each other during our cancer journeys! Thank you for supporting this book and believing in it. I love you both, and I am excited that we can all now say we are cancer-free.

Grandmere (yet another survivor): I know you are no longer with us, but I know that you are watching from heaven, proud of me. I know that you would approve of the person I have become, and I appreciate all of the wisdom and strength you instilled in me before you left us. I miss you and love you very much.

H.P., L.T., J.C., E.W., K.M., D.L., E.G.: Thank you all so very much for being there for me, especially during my cancer journey. I cannot thank you enough for your love and support. Please know that my friendship with each and every one of you means the world to me. I love you all.

The list goes on. It's truly impossible to name every person who has reached out and sent well wishes and prayers my way. Please know that I am grateful for each and every one of you. You know who you are. You have all brought the biggest smile to my face, and I appreciate it more than you know. Thank you.

Preface

This book was very difficult for me to write. Although I wrote the bulk of it throughout my journey, I continued to work on it months after my treatments were over. I needed to go back and finalize my story, ensuring that every word and detail was on point. This forced me to reread everything and relive the awful memories. Each time, as I bawled my eyes out, I would sit there in devastation and ask myself, "Did I really go through this?"

Since the very first day this journey began, I knew I needed to document it. I didn't do this for myself; I did it for every single person who would, unfortunately, be diagnosed with cancer. I felt very strongly in my spirit that I needed to write this book to help, encourage, and inspire every cancer patient who needed some advice and guidance. I knew that, as intelligent and helpful oncologists and nurses are, they can only tell you so much unless they themselves have undergone cancer treatment. Unfortunately, oncologists and nurses who have never been diagnosed with cancer have a very limited scope of what they can tell you. Yes, they know the side effects of chemotherapy, and they are well-aware of what their patients deal with. The problem, however, was that I had to learn so many things on my own, without ever being warned about them. That's why I wrote this book: to document my journey and give cancer patients a heads-up about what to expect, offering insight and advice based on my experience.

I pray that this book helps anyone going through cancer. I am incredibly proud of what I have written, and I hope it touches anyone who reads it.

This book is raw and uncensored. Nothing is sugar-coated or embellished.

This is my story. This is my miracle.

Introduction

Cancer. Six letters and two syllables. Who knew such a small word could cause so much damage? I guarantee that anyone you talk to knows someone who has been diagnosed with cancer or has gone through it themselves. What in the world is going on these days? Are we getting cancer because of the foods we eat? Because of the chemical-laden body products we put on our skin? Because of our lifestyle choices? Genetics? Bad luck?

Regardless of the *why*, I want to help with the *how*. How can we conquer such an ugly disease while wearing smiles on our faces and having good attitudes? How can we go through this journey feeling empowered and inspired, rather than perpetually sad and angry? How can we stay positive during this difficult time?

Here is one thing I have learned: Your attitude is *everything*. If you have the right attitude during your treatment, it makes a huge difference. Yes, there are going to be days when you want to crawl up in a ball and cry—and that's okay—but overall, you need to stay strong mentally. You need to have a positive mental attitude, or PMA. Your PMA will not only make things easier on you but will cause you to heal faster than you ever thought possible.

You're going to conquer cancer, and it's as simple as that. Those negative thoughts, sleepless nights, and everything in between stop right here. You are not a victim. You are not weak. You are not hopeless. You are strong and confident. You are powerful, positive, and a warrior. You are going to fight this head on, and nothing is going to stop you. You are the ultimate badass.

Before I divulge what happened on this day, let me start by saying I am the healthiest person I know. I take care of my body like nobody's business. I take my vitamins, use organic body products, eat organic produce, drink alkaline water, and spend my time researching vitamins and supplements like it's my job. Health and wellness have always been my passion, and I have been regretting the fact that I did not become a nutritionist. In short, I have always been obsessed with being healthy.

Six months to a year before this, my sister had noticed a bump in my sternum area. Me, being completely stubborn and anti-doctors, had shrugged it off and paid no attention to it. In April of 2015, I had begun noticing that when I would drink any sort of alcoholic beverage, I would get horrible pains up and down my arms as well as in my chest. Again, I never saw a doctor about this because it had been hard for me to find a primary care physician that I truly trusted since moving to Colorado seven years before. The few PCP's I had seen in my time in Colorado had either been extremely rude or had no idea what they were doing, so I tried to avoid doctors as much as I could.

On this day, I went to Urgent Care to try to get this bump figured out. Lately, it had looked like it was getting bigger and bigger, and it was honestly beginning to scare me. I had named it Billy Bob. Billy Bob Bump was his full name.

On a side note: another reason I never thought twice about this was because my late grandmother had a bump on her sternum, and she lived until 87, so my initial thought was *Maybe it's a good-luck bump?*

At the Urgent Care, I got some X-rays done of my chest. The doctor saw the X-rays and immediately asked if I thought it was the C word: cancer. Me? Cancer? Absolutely not. No way. I was 28 years old and took good care of my body. NOPE. Cancer wasn't even an option. The thought of it was absolutely absurd to me. The doctor asked me if I had any pain at all. Nope, I felt great and healthy all the time. No joke. ALL. THE. TIME. I've never even gotten the flu, for crying out loud.

I left the Urgent Care and was so disturbed at the fact that this doctor, after seeing an X-ray, would jump the gun and already start tossing the cancer word around. Like, are you kidding me right now? *Typical doctor*, I thought.

January 25, 2016

On my way home from work tonight, I received a call from the Urgent Care doctor. He informed me that the radiologist who had looked at my X-rays was "concerned." I was in the middle of driving home and was super freaked out, obviously. "Concerned" is never a good word coming from the doctor. I was instructed that I needed to get a CT scan done, and then a biopsy. I immediately called my best friend, Heather, after I got off the phone with the doctor. My heart was pounding, and tears were streaming down my face.

That night, my mind was flooded with a million thoughts: *What is going on with my body? What the heck is in my chest? Am I going to be okay?* Because of my strong faith in God, I tried to quiet my mind and started praying relentlessly. This was by far the scariest thing to ever happen to me, but something inside me knew I was going to be fine.

This was all happening just a few months after my 22-year-old sister had been diagnosed with melanoma, the deadliest and most aggressive form of skin cancer. During the summer, she had developed what looked like a bug bite on the back of her leg. Because it had not healed right away, she had decided to see a dermatologist, who had quickly diagnosed her with melanoma. She then needed to have two separate surgeries and also begin a treatment called Yervoy. I will get into this in greater detail a little later on, but because I can't help myself, I need to take this opportunity to say that if you use a tanning bed, stop immediately! You are literally paying to get cancer. If you really want to be tan, you can use organic self-tanner or go get a spray tan. When you use regular tanning beds, you are doing a lot of damage to your body—so stop. Just stop.

That night, it seemed like suddenly, chaos had started happening out of nowhere. The unknown is incredibly scary, but I managed to get some sleep and did my best to stay positive.

January 26, 2016

While I was at work, I received a phone call from one of the staff at the Urgent Care. He was a sweetheart and had assisted me when I had gone there a couple of days before. "I want to give you the number to the cancer center," he told me. WHAT THE HECK?! I hadn't even had a CT scan or biopsy done yet, and already I was being told to contact a cancer center? "We are thinking you might have bone cancer," he stated.

Are you freaking kidding me right now?! Can everyone just calm down for a hot minute? There I was, in my office at work, having someone tell me that I might possibly have bone cancer.

"Write this word down," he instructed. He then went on to spell "osteosarcoma" for me – bone cancer. I couldn't believe what was happening.

I took the cancer center's number down and laughed it off. *I do not have cancer*, I kept thinking.

Later that day, because I guess everyone was so damn eager to diagnose me before I had even had a biopsy done, I received a call from the cancer center. I let it go straight to voicemail.

January 29, 2016

Today, I had my very first CT scan done. Both my mom and friend Je'nean went with me for support. The nurse called me back and asked me to change into a gown.

The actual process wasn't as bad as I had thought it would be. The nurse asked me all sorts of questions. "How long have you noticed this bump in your chest?"

"Between six months to a year," I explained.

"Any pain?"

"No pain whatsoever."

"What did the doctors say this could be?" she asked.

"They think it's canc—the C word," I hesitantly stated.

"Oh dear, well let's hope it's not that!"

Yes, honey, from your mouth to God's ears.

As the scan was performed, I lay very still, even though I was shaking a little from being nervous. A loud voice spoke through the CT scan machine. "Breathe in," it instructed. I held my breath for a moment, and then the voice came back. "Breathe out."

Before I knew it, the scan was over. The nurse explained to me that the radiologist would be looking it over soon and I would get a call as soon as they heard something. Unsure of how to feel, I walked out of the building with my mom and Je'nean and tried to forget about everything.

That night, my mom and I were at my apartment, waiting for the doctor to call me with the CT scan results. We spent time praying and asking God for good results. We read scriptures specifically for healing. We felt good about everything, although yes, I was still freaking out in my head.

After we had been praying for about fifteen minutes, the Urgent Care doctor called me. He sounded somber. He couldn't get his words together. "So, Jen, um, I have your results."

Okay, spit it out!

"Well, this, this just doesn't look good. Both the radiologist and I have never seen anything like this before. Um. I just want you to prepare for the worst."

My heart stopped. I was too shocked to cry or do anything. After I hung up the phone with the doctor, my mom and I prayed again. This time, we gave the issue to God and knew He was completely in control. The hard part, though, was knowing God was in control and then still worrying about it. I knew I couldn't do both; I either trusted God or I didn't. I knew I needed to trust Him, no matter what the outcome was. And no matter what the outcome was, I knew I was going to be okay.

February 4, 2016

I was scheduled to have a biopsy done early this morning. I was supposed to be out of the hospital by 11 a.m. The plan was that the doctors would review my CT scan results, which were given to them on a CD. After the doctors had reviewed the CT scan, the biopsy would be performed. As I was lying in a gown in the hospital bed, waiting to be wheeled into the surgery room, a radiologist and nurse came into my room.

"So, the CT scan CD we were given is completely blank, so we weren't able to see what's going on. We need to do another CT scan this morning before you can get the biopsy."

Annoyed, I bit my tongue.

The radiologist continued, "I'm sure you've read your reports thus far. We're thinking this is lymphoma. This is serious stuff."

Um, *excuse me?* What reports could I have read? I'm not a doctor, so even if I had seen any reports, I would have had no idea what I'd be reading! And *lymphoma?* What the heck? I didn't even know what it was, exactly, except for some form of cancer. First I had been told bone cancer, and now lymphoma? Why in the world was everyone making all of these assumptions before I had even had a biopsy done?

And then I realized that *this* was why I avoided doctors like the plague. So many of them could be cold and matter-of-fact, forgetting that we are humans and not robots.

I couldn't even respond because I was crying so hard. The radiologist was emotionless. I couldn't believe what was happening.

I had to redo the CT scan, wait for the results, and *then* get the biopsy done. The room I got the biopsy done in was actually pretty cozy. It was dimly lit and very relaxing.

They numbed my chest area and took some tissue from Billy Bob. It was at that time that I was informed that I had an approximately 10-centimeter mass in my chest, sitting on my heart. It wasn't affecting my heart in any way, but it was obviously very concerning. Turns out, Billy Bob was trying to kill me.

After the biopsy was complete, I was wheeled back into my hospital room, and that's when I met an angel. She was a nurse named Valerie, and she turned everything around for me.

Valerie oozed compassion and love. As I was lying in the bed, speaking to Valerie, she noticed the bump in my chest and simply thought it was swollen from having the biopsy done. Nope, it wasn't swollen from that. It was just a big ol' mass in my chest. I tried to explain this to Valerie as tears poured out of my eyes uncontrollably.

We began talking, and she asked what was going on with me. In between sobs, I informed her that the doctor suspected I may have lymphoma. Valerie grabbed my hand and looked at me with an unbelievable amount of love. Then she shut the door and said, "I want to tell you something."

She told me a story about how her ex-husband had had lymphoma many, many years before. "Look," she said to me, "if it is what they're saying it is, the good news is that lymphoma is curable—*curable*—and the survival rate is very high. Treatments have come such a long way, too. So try not to worry."

It was because of Valerie that I walked out of the hospital feeling calm as could be. It was the craziest feeling, actually, because you'd think I'd be flipping out over the fact that I could possibly have cancer. In that moment, however, I knew that no matter what, I was going to be okay. Like, it wasn't even a second thought. My faith was intact, and so was my mental clarity. Good thing for that, though, because little did I know that this was only the beginning of my journey.

February 9, 2016

My dad and I walked into the cancer center in Denver so I could get my biopsy results. Something about this building reminded me of the older buildings in my hometown in New Jersey. For a split second, I was provided with an ounce of comfort. It didn't last long, though. I just kept telling myself, *I do not have cancer; I do not have cancer*, over and over in my head. My heart was pounding. I had never been so nervous in my entire life.

This was occurring as my mom was rushing to my sister's side in Tulsa. My sister was back in the hospital, sick as a dog thanks to Yervoy, and my mom needed to be with her, so today, I was just with my dad. Because we were all so confident that there was nothing seriously wrong with me, we were all in agreement that my mom should definitely be with my sister instead of at the cancer center with me.

Finally, after what felt like an eternity, a nurse called me back. She took my vitals and my height and weight. Then they stuck my dad and me in the room to meet the oncologist. I swear, it felt like we were waiting for the doctor for an eternity. I got more anxious by the minute, armpits damp, heart pounding. I made the mistake of reading flyers posted on the wall. One read, "Are you anxious about beginning life after chemotherapy? Come to our free seminar." I kept taking deep breaths and fidgeting with my fingers. The wait was stressing me out like no other.

Finally, the physician's assistant came into the room and introduced herself. She seemed nice, and I began to feel somewhat calm again. She sat down and asked me, "So, have they gone over your treatment plan with you yet?" That's when everything around me stood still.

"Um... well, no one has told me anything yet. I don't even know what's going on!" I frantically began spewing.

The room got silent, and the PA's expression got awkward. "Oh, um, well no one told you?"

"TOLD ME WHAT?"

After a brief pause, the PA declared, "Well, you have what they call Hodgkin's lymphoma..."

I didn't hear the rest of what she said because everything around me went black. Tears immediately poured out of my eyes, dampening my entire face, running down my neck, soaking my sweater. Eye makeup smeared. I tried to catch my breath but had difficulty doing so. My dad was next to me and I knew he wanted to cry, too, but he needed to be strong for me.

So, this was what it was like to have your worst fear come true.

My heart broke for my mom and dad. They were officially the parents of two daughters who currently had cancer. One daughter was rough enough, but two? My head was spinning.

I finally composed myself, trying to listen to what the PA was telling me. She told me what Valerie had told me: Lymphoma is curable and the survival rate is high. That was comforting, but still… *it was freaking cancer!*

Moments later, I met my oncologist. I will call him Dr. J.

I instantly got good vibes from Dr. J. He had a very kind face and had compassion in his eyes. I got a sense that he really cared about his patients and that he was good at his job. Dr. J apologized for the confusion. He had been under the impression that I had already received my diagnosis from the doctor I had seen at the Urgent Care. He went on to say, "Lymphoma is probably the best cancer to have," since the survival rate is very high. Although I'd prefer not to have cancer, I guess having the "best" kind was uplifting. I then learned exactly what lymphoma was. It's cancer of the lymphatic system.

Dr. J answered all of my questions and made me feel comfortable with everything. As it turns out, those pains from alcoholic drinks were actually because of Hodgkin's. Crazy, right?

I was then informed that I would need to begin chemotherapy. Dr. J predicted that I would need anywhere from four to six cycles of chemo, each cycle consisting of two treatments. Treatments would be done every other week, meaning I would be done with treatment by the summer.

"Okay," I said, "here's the thing: I am not going to lose my hair from chemo, and I am not going to miss my best friend's wedding at the end of March in Jersey. Those are my only concerns." Because I had already been told that certain chemo treatments did not cause complete hair loss, I felt confident that I would keep my hair. He told me to buy a wig, just in case, but that hair loss varies for all patients who are doing the treatment I would be doing. Dr. J also let me know that I could schedule my chemo around the wedding so I would be able to attend.

On the drive home, I was at peace. My dad helped me feel calm, too. We went out for ribs that night. "Screw it," I said. "I spent my whole life taking care of myself and I still got cancer. Let's chow down on some fatty ribs."

After dinner, I spoke to my boyfriend on the phone. I knew I needed to have a positive attitude about this, and I knew that I needed to have a good sense of humor, so I decided to try out some cancer pick-up lines. "Hey baby," I said to him, "do chicks with cancer who have bumps in their chest turn you on? If so, I'm the girl for you." I knew that the only way I could get through this cancer journey was by having three things: faith, humor, and a positive attitude. I had all three, and I intended on keeping it that way.

Instead of the chemo being administered through an IV in your arm, they began doing it through what is called a port. A port is surgically put into your chest area and connects to your heart. It looks freaky because you can see it poking through your skin. It's just... *so weird*.

I needed to have my port put in today. I wasn't going to be put under general anesthesia but would be given the "twilight." Because I'd never had any medical issues before, I had no idea what to expect, and needless to say, I was incredibly nervous.

I sat in the hospital room in a sexy hospital gown and waited for the nurse to come in, hoping it would be Valerie. A different nurse came in, however, and began prepping me. When she was done, she was about to leave the room for a minute.

Before she left, I asked her if Valerie was working that day, and the nurse told me yes. "Could you do me a favor and just let her know I said hello, and tell her I said thank you?"

The nurse smiled. "Of course."

Moments later, Valerie popped her head into the room. "A little birdie told me you were here again."

That's when I completely lost it and broke down. Just seeing Valerie's face was enough to bring me to tears. She came over and gave me a hug and kiss, and asked what was going on. When I told her, she offered me more encouragement and told me to give her an update when I was cancer-free.

I got that feeling of calmness again once I had seen her. It was amazing that God put her in my life.

A new nurse came into the room and introduced himself to me as Chris. He cracked a few jokes to calm my nerves and began wheeling me to the operating room. He continued to joke around with me, and I found it impossible to not feel better.

Once we got to the operating room, I was introduced to the radiologist who would be doing my port procedure. This radiologist was different from the emotionless one who had traumatized me before my biopsy. I instantly liked this new radiologist. He had a very kind smile, and I got a sense of genuineness from him. He explained to me that three years before, he had gone through lymphoma himself. The fact that he was totally fine now was comforting. I also found out shortly after that, that one of the nurses who would be assisting with the port procedure was going through chemo for lymphoma. *What the hell is going on?* I thought. *Why is it so common?*

When the procedure was about to begin, I was transferred from my hospital bed to the operating room bed. Chris informed me that he was going to begin administering the twilight cocktail. Soon after, I began feeling really good, almost like I was drunk, which was a delightful feeling since I hadn't been able to enjoy any alcohol for almost a year.

The doctor numbed my chest area so I wouldn't feel anything, and he also put a sheet up by my neck—kind of like what they do when you get a C-section. I had my eyes closed the whole time, but I was still conscious. The only thing I remember saying was, "This medicine is great. Can I take some home with me?"

Before I knew it, the procedure was over. I started talking to the nurse who had lymphoma. She looked great. "You still have your hair!" I pointed out in my sedated state.

"Yup!" she replied. "It's fragile and it breaks pretty easily, but I'm not going to lose it all." Knowing there was a chance I wouldn't lose my hair during chemo was a humongous relief. One of the first things I had thought of—actually, who am I kidding? *The* first thing I thought of— after I had been told I would need chemo was hair loss. Just think of how traumatizing it is to lose all your hair! My hair was super-long, going all the way down my back. I had grown up with many people telling me that my hair was one of my best features. If I were to lose my hair, then what? The thought of it gave me so much anxiety, but now it appeared as if there was hope that I wouldn't go bald.

I was taken back to the hospital room for recovery. The twilight cocktail, sadly, wore off, and I was feeling back to normal in no time. What wasn't normal, however, was the foreign object in my body. I could barely stand the sight of it. It looked like a baby alien trying to claw its way out of my chest. I just couldn't deal with it.

Later that night, I began realizing that maybe it still hadn't hit me yet that this whole cancer thing was a reality for me. I was doing my best to stay positive and not let anything get me down. I was praying harder than usual and continued to feel a sense of peace. Was I crazy for not spending my time crying uncontrollably and worrying about my health? I think it just meant that my faith was unshakeable. One thing I knew was that this journey would be rough. I didn't, however, realize exactly how rough.

"I want this thing out of me," I told someone, referring to the port. It was just too creepy for me to deal with, and on top of that, I had been experiencing some major discomfort. It felt like the port was twitching. The more I freaked out about it, the worse it got. I tried to remain calm, but it was just so weird.

I also started to begin feeling like an invalid. I couldn't really do much with my right side, the side my port was on, because it was pretty sore. I could barely lift my arm when putting on a shirt. Little things like cleaning and showering were difficult, and that difficulty was becoming a nuisance. Luckily, I had been told that within a week, I would begin feeling better.

Having a foreign object inside of me was just the creepiest feeling, though. How would I ever get used to this? Aside from having this hideous-looking alien inside of me, I needed to finally tell my mom and sister about what was going on with me. They were both still in Tulsa. My sister was back home from the hospital, feeling better, and until this point, I had been keeping them both in the dark about my diagnosis. My dad and I had agreed to wait to tell them the news until after my sister was on the mend, because I needed my mom to focus on helping my sister get better, and I didn't need my sister having additional stress, which could hinder her healing process.

I decided to video chat with them to tell them the news. Before I told them, I explained why I hadn't told them right away. Then I blurted out, "I have Hodgkin's lymphoma."

As they both began crying, I assured them that my prognosis was good and that I would be just fine. It was a very emotional time. Seeing their faces through my computer, not being able to hug them and tell them that everything would be okay, broke my heart. "Danielle, we are Jersey girls," I joked with my sister. "A little cancer can't defeat us!"

My sister seemed to be on the mend at this point, and now it would be my turn to begin my journey. I would begin chemo in ten days. *Please, God, let's just get this over with,* I prayed.

February 15, 2016

Today, I needed to have a PET scan done. This is slightly different from a CT scan, as PET scans are able to detect cancer in the body. Unsure of how to feel, I tried to do my best to relax. I mean, I was already well-aware of the fact that I had lymphoma, so having this scan done wasn't anything to be nervous about.

I was at a different cancer center location, closer to my apartment. This would now be the primary location for my chemo and appointments.

As I met with one of the nurses, I looked around the cancer center. Plenty of nurses were scattered about, tending to their patients. Seeing them, I was struck with sadness because I realized that all of these nurses were busy because their patients had cancer. This whole cancer center was funded because of this awful disease, a disease that takes the lives of so many people each day. It was absolutely terrible, but I needed to refocus my energy on positive things, so I came to the realization that this cancer center was helping the patients become cancer-free. The nurses, the doctors, the staff... all of them had their part in helping all of the cancer patients who walked through the doors. I felt better after coming to that realization.

After that brief wave of sadness passed over me, I was injected with some radioactive dye and was told to listen to some music and be as still as possible for approximately a half hour. I was put in a recliner and dozed off until the nurse gave me a bottled water to chug. Shortly after I drank the water, the PET scan began.

As I lay on the narrow bed, I immediately started feeling a tad claustrophobic. I kept my eyes tightly shut the entire time as I moved back and forth in the machine. At one point, the bed stopped moving and stayed in one place for what felt like an eternity. Too afraid to open my eyes, I started listening for any sign of human life in the room. Nothing. I began convincing myself that the nurses had forgotten about me. Perhaps they had gone to grab a cup of coffee and chat about their non-cancer lives. Perhaps they had decided to go on a shopping spree. Whatever they had decided, I was convinced that I had been forgotten, left behind. At that point, it was just me, myself, and Billy Bob—Billy Bob, that bastard.

In reality, though, I knew I hadn't been forgotten about. Shortly after a brief moment of panic, I began moving back and forth again. And finally, *finally*, the PET scan concluded and I was able to get out of the machine, unharmed.

The rest of the day went smoothly. I went to work and was able to function as if everything was perfectly normal.

My dad and I went to a "chemo teach class" today. In this class, a nurse meets with you to go over everything you need to know about chemotherapy.

When I got to the cancer center, a nurse greeted me and took my dad and me back into a small conference room. She had a big folder full of papers. She didn't waste any time. She explained that my chemo regimen was called ABVD, and she went over all of the possible side effects: nausea, constipation, diarrhea, fatigue, mouth sores, dry skin, anxiety, infertility, neuropathy, etc. The list went on and on. She also explained that the B part of my treatment—bleomycin—could possibly cause issues with my lungs. Isn't that fantastic? She said that during my first treatment, they would start off by administering just a small dose and see if I had a reaction. If I didn't, then I was good to go.

"So, is this going to cause lung cancer down the road?" I asked. The nurse said no, but if anything, it would cause shortness of breath or breathing issues. *No big deal.*

I was surprised that the nurse hadn't yet mentioned anything about hair. Because I knew two people who hadn't lost their hair during treatment for lymphoma (that nurse from my port placement, as well as a family friend), I was confident that I wouldn't lose mine. When I explained this to the nurse, she looked me dead in the eyes and gently said, "You're going to lose your hair."

Everything stood still. Cue the water works. In that moment, I was more freaked out about being bald than having cancer. What was wrong with this picture?

My dad tried to calm me down. "Jen, it's hair. It will grow back."

He was absolutely right, it would grow back, but the thought of being bald was terrifying to me. *Terrifying*.

"After your second treatment, you will lose your hair," the nurse declared. Not only were those words devastating in themselves, but the timing couldn't be worse. On March 25, two weeks and two days after my second treatment, would be the wedding I had told Dr. J about. I was going to be a bridesmaid in it, and I would be with my boyfriend for the trip. There's no way in hell I would let him see me bald.

It sounded incredibly vain, but I immediately started thinking of how ugly I would look and feel if I lost all my hair. And my eyelashes. And my eyebrows. What would be left of me? I would have no identity whatsoever. I could try to wear makeup, and maybe get some false lashes, but I would still need to take them off at the end of the day. How could I look at myself in the mirror at night?

Both the nurse and my dad tried to calm me down and bring me back to the session to discuss some other issues. As hung up as I was about the hair thing, I needed to pay attention to the rest of the information.

The nurse gave me four prescriptions: one for anxiety and nausea, and to help me sleep; one for nausea during the day; one for numbing cream to apply to my port prior to chemo; and one for a cranial pros-thesis, or wig. I bit my lip and tried not to cry again.

"Wigs could get expensive," the nurse explained, "so we need to give you a prescription so your insurance can help pay for it."

I walked out of the cancer center feeling like I had just been beaten up. The hair thing weighed heavily on my mind. I tried reasoning with myself: *Okay, what's worse—losing your hair or your life?*

I needed to try to stop being ridiculous.

February 21, 2016

Over the weekend, I made a quick trip to Jersey to attend my friend Lisa's bachelorette party. Her fiancé wanted to surprise her by having me fly out, so he had purchased my ticket so I could spend some time with her.

The bachelorette party wasn't anything too crazy. No strippers. No wild, drunken nights. It was a nice evening with some really great people. And the biggest blessing of all was the fact that I was able to spend time with Lisa before I started chemo in a few days.

As I was waiting for my flight to take me back to Denver, I began thinking about something. When we are on an airplane, we automati-cally develop a trust in the pilot. Sometimes we don't even see the pilot before or after the flight, but we know the pilot is there all along, doing his or her job. When there's turbulence during the flight, we trust that the pilot knows how to handle this and keep us safe. We know that the pilot has had special training to prepare for all situations and is in control.

In the same sense, we should have that same trust in God. We need to realize that God is in complete control of every aspect of our lives. When life has its turbulence, we have to stay calm, because God is with us, even though we can't see Him. Like with the pilot, we need to relax and believe that God will keep us safe and get us through the ups and downs.

With that thought, I closed my eyes and fell asleep during the flight. I knew that in just a few short days, when I began chemo, there would be some turbulence. The good thing, though, was knowing that God is the ultimate pilot.

February 23, 2016

Here's the thing: Just because you like your doctor doesn't mean you can't get a second opinion. If you have recently been diagnosed with cancer, I think the best thing to do is always get a second opinion. This way, you will never have any regrets or second guesses.

This is just what I did. It wasn't because I didn't trust Dr. J. That wasn't it at all. I knew that he had my best interest in mind and was doing his job, but I wanted to make absolutely sure that I couldn't opt for radiation in lieu of chemo.

I met with a different oncologist at a different cancer center in Denver, just to be on the safe side. At first, I wasn't crazy about this oncologist when he walked in the door. It's incredible how first impressions are everything. He had a very stern look on his face and simply said, "Hi," when he walked in. He was very cold and was nothing like Dr. J. As we began talking, however, he seemed to warm up a bit.

This oncologist explained that he agreed with Dr. J about my treatment plan. He said that for my specific diagnosis, anywhere I went, they would tell me I needed the same chemo treatment: ABVD. I didn't have just the tumor in my chest. The PET scan had shown that I also had cancer in my lymph nodes underneath my armpits and near my neck, so not even surgery was an option. I also learned that for lymphoma, the cancer can never be removed via surgery, because there's a good chance surgery could cause the cancer to spread.

Even though this wasn't the news I was hoping for, I knew that now, I would never have any regrets about not getting a second opinion. Through this process, you need to be your own advocate. You need to do your own research and be prepared to ask a lot of questions. My issue was that I was too fearful to begin researching Hodgkin's lymphoma. The Internet is a scary place, and you're always going to find people with all different kinds of opinions, some good and some bad. And then you might come across statistics that don't look good, or side effects that you didn't think were possible. But it's necessary to find websites that are trustworthy so you can do the proper research. Looking at blogs written by cancer patients, for example, may not be the best idea, because some people are going to have bad experiences. The things written on those blogs aren't always uplifting. They might mention recurrences or secondary cancers, and that will completely freak you out. My point is to use your best judgment when looking up your type of cancer online.

The next day, I would begin chemo. I really didn't know how I was feeling, mainly because I didn't quite know what to expect. All of those possible side effects seemed really scary. I knew, though, that I needed to stay strong and continue having faith that I would be okay no matter what.

February 24, 2016

And so it began. This was the day of my first treatment. I woke up feeling fine, not too nervous or anything. I ate a healthy breakfast, put the numbing cream on my port, and headed out the door. My parents accompanied me, and I was grateful that they were there with me.

After I walked into the cancer center with my parents, I checked in with the receptionist and waited to be called back. A nurse greeted me and took me back to take my vitals and weight. Then I needed to go get blood work done. They would poke me in my port to draw blood, and then leave this little tube sticking out of my port until chemo began. Then they would simply use that tube to administer the chemo through. What I would soon realize is that one of the worst parts about the chemo process, in my opinion, is the gross saline taste you get in your mouth. After they do the blood work, they flush your port to clean it, and for whatever reason, you can taste the saline in your mouth. The trick is to always suck on some candy as they do it. Then it becomes somewhat tolerable.

As I was getting my blood drawn, a woman sitting next to me was going through the same thing. There was something about her calm demeanor that made me believe she was a pro at this. She was very pretty and was probably in her forties. Here's what caught my attention: She still had her hair. And a lot of it, I might add. I could tell it wasn't a wig, either. I had absolutely no idea what cancer she had, but the fact that she still had her hair gave me hope. It instantly made me feel better.

After my blood work, I went into a room to meet with Dr. J. He asked how I was doing, and I couldn't complain, except for the hair thing. Dr. J explained that they need to warn patients of all of the possible side effects. I was just eager to get this over and done with. The faster I got in, the faster I could get out.

My parents and I were instructed to enter the large chemo room and sit wherever we wanted, so we walked in, found some chairs, and waited for a nurse. All of the patients got to sit in comfortable recliners. *I was the youngest patient in the room.*

I still wasn't nervous. In fact, I was cracking some jokes with my parents and acting as if I was spending a day at the beach. I knew I needed to stay positive to get through this. I just kept telling myself that soon, this would all be a memory. Even though I was currently a cancer patient, I sure as hell wasn't going to be one forever. *This is temporary*, I told myself.

A nurse came over to me and introduced herself, then explained how the whole process worked. First, they would administer the anti-nausea medicine, and then they would begin administering the chemo. Because it was my first time, they would need to ensure I didn't have a reaction to the bleomycin.

After administering the anti-nausea medicine, they administered a small dose of bleomycin. I waited about fifteen minutes and felt completely fine. That's when the nurse knew my body had accepted it, so she finished administering the rest.

"Did they warn you about hair thinning?" she asked. I explained to her that I kept hearing different things and that I heard that I could either keep my hair or lose all of it. The nurse was a little confused when I told her that and said, "All of my patients who are on your chemo regimen only experience hair thinning."

This was an incredible relief. Luckily, my hair was super thick, so even if it thinned, it probably wouldn't be very noticeable. I felt like the weight of the world was off my shoulders. She instantly lifted my spirits. I couldn't keep my excitement to myself; I frantically began texting my friends to tell them the good news.

As I hung out with poison pumping into my body, my parents and I struck up a conversation with a couple sitting next to us. Their names were John and Pam. John had non-Hodgkin's, and this was his last treatment. He was kind enough to give me some tips. For example, he told me to stay on top of the nausea medication. If the instructions said to take it every six hours, he told me, I should take it every five hours. He said the worst thing you could do is not be on top of it, because that's when the nausea will creep up on you and then come at you full force.

During my conversation with John and Pam, an elderly woman who had just finished up her round of chemo walked over to me. "What's your name, sweetheart?" she asked. I told her, and she shook my hand and said she would be praying for me. What I would quickly learn was that now, I was part of this community. We cancer patients were bonded—by this terrible disease and by this chemo we were receiving. We were all there for one another, and despite the fact that we were total strangers, we could immediately bond over what we were going through. It was a pretty cool feeling.

The whole chemo session was only about three hours long for me. That's when the nurse came over to me and took the tube out of my port, telling me I was all done. Talking to John and Pam had definitely helped the time pass, and I was grateful for that. I said good-bye to them, and John and I wished each other well.

I walked out of the cancer center feeling totally fine. Then I made my first mistake, which no one had warned me about. Here's something crucial for everyone to know who is going through chemo: the foods that you eat during and right after chemo may very easily become foods you will never, ever want to touch again. I don't know if it's because you will begin associating those foods with chemo and/or nausea, but regardless, be mindful of that.

Right after chemo, I went to an eatery that I really enjoyed. I ordered one of my favorite salads and a green juice. This meal was one I had eaten quite a few times in the past. Little did I know that soon after, just the *thought* of this particular meal would make me want to throw up. No joke. Soon after, I realized that salads and green juices would go under my list of "bad foods" that I wouldn't be able to stomach for a very, very long time.

After I ate lunch, I popped into the local health food shop for a few things. During my time there, I started feeling slightly sick. I guess I had reached my limit. Here's another tip: Listen to your body. Listening to your body is important because during chemo, you are fragile. You are having poison pumped into your body, and it is killing *everything*—the good and the bad—in your body. During this time, you really need to go easy and be kind to yourself. A cancer survivor I had met once told me, "Don't try to play the hero." If you don't feel well enough to do something, don't do it. If you are unable to do something, the people around you—your family, friends, bosses, etc.—will understand. And if they don't, you should probably rethink whether you want them in your life.

After the health food shop, I spent the night at my parents' house. I had taken the next day off work, but to my surprise, I was able to go to work on Friday, just two days after my first treatment. The nausea during this time wasn't terrible. I mean, I felt crappy, but not to the point of wanting to throw up my guts. Thankfully, on Friday, I was able to get work done, and I felt pretty good. I thought, *Wow, this chemo thing isn't as bad as I thought it would be.*

I guess I should also take this time to point out that my bosses, Dave and Mike, were supportive and amazing when I told them about my health issue. They told me not to worry about work and that the number-one priority was me getting better. They weren't going to penalize me for taking days off for chemo or doctor appointments; I was so relieved that I wanted to cry. My plan was to simply take Wednesdays off for chemo and then attempt to work from home on Thursdays. I knew that if I was too sick to work from home, though, that my bosses would be very understanding and I didn't need to worry. Seriously, I couldn't ask for better people to work for.

Here's another thing you need to think about when you are diagnosed with cancer: choosing whether you want to tell everyone. Obviously, all my friends and family knew. I had amazing people in my life, and after I was diagnosed, I was overwhelmed by the love and support by those around me. When it came to the people I worked with, however, I chose to tell only four people out of an office of fourteen. I obviously needed to tell my bosses, and I also told my friend at work, Kaitlynn. And because I trusted them, I knew they wouldn't tell anyone else. I didn't want the whole office knowing, for a few reasons. I guess the first was because I was a very private person and I didn't like when attention was on me. I didn't feel it was necessary for me to make an announcement at work, like, "Hey, everybody, I have cancer!" That just wasn't me.

The second reason was because—let's face it—sometimes people really don't know how to act around someone who is going through cancer if they aren't very close with that person. The last thing I wanted to do was make anyone feel uncomfortable or awkward.

The last and most important reason was because when I was at work, I wasn't Jen the cancer patient; I was simply Jen the paralegal. I can't tell you how good it felt to just go to work and be "normal." Because the majority of the office had no clue what I was going through, I was treated like a normal, average, healthy person. And because I was treated that way, my mind was relaxed (for the most part) and sometimes I would actually forget about what I was dealing with in my personal life.

Maybe you don't have a choice about telling your coworkers about what you're going through, and that's fine. Or maybe you are fine with everyone knowing. If you are, great! It really just comes down to your level of comfort.

One more thing: The people who do know about what you are going through are always going to be giving you unsolicited advice ("Stay away from sugar, because cancer feeds off sugar; make sure you take Vitamins X, Y, and Z, because those will help kill cancer cells; and so on). People mean well, really, but when you are dealing with the horrible side effects of chemo, taking that sort of advice is easier said than done. Sometimes it's really difficult to stay away from sugary foods because, let's face it, those foods may be the only foods you can tolerate during chemo. A lot of foods that you used to enjoy are soon going to be foods you can't. Listen to your body and do the best you can. If certain healthy foods make you feel nauseous, stay away from them, even if they are sugar-free, gluten-free, dairy-free, non-GMO, and vegan. As I mentioned already, just listen to your body and eat whatever foods don't make you feel like you're going to throw up.

February 27, 2016

I woke up on this morning with horrible pains in my chest. I wasn't sure what was happening, but I assumed it was my port giving me some trouble. I woke up early and then went back to sleep until 11 a.m., which was unheard of for me. I always woke up around 7 a.m. on the weekends.

I couldn't stay in bed past 11, though, because I had plans with my aunt Denise to go wig shopping, even though I was praying that I wouldn't ever need to wear one.

After I met my aunt, we drove to the wig shop. We looked at all the different kinds there. There were so many to choose from! The owner of the wig shop, who had gone through cancer herself many years before, helped me try on a bunch of different wigs. My hair was long and blonde, and she showed me wigs that looked exactly like my own hair.

After trying on the first wig, I lost it. Seeing myself in a wig automatically made me feel, for the first time, like a cancer patient. I think that's when it started to really hit me. As I stared at myself in the mirror, I simply couldn't keep it together.

My aunt was there to hug me and comfort me. I felt just awful, but after those brief moments of sadness, I tried making the best of the situation. I started thinking how, if I did lose my hair, it would be fun to have a bunch of different styles of wigs, and they could be my alter egos. For example, I would get a short dark-brown wig and name her Tanya. Tanya was pretty slutty and liked to stay out late, partying in downtown Denver. I would also have a long red wig named Angelica. Angelica was the sexy bookworm who enjoyed book clubs and intellectual conversations. My point is, how you look at things is important. Even though what you're going through sucks and is very serious, you need to try to keep a good perspective on things.

My number-one goal was trying to find humor even during the storm. Sometimes, I felt like I was in the midst of a terrible storm, but then I'd think of something funny and would just begin cracking up. Whether it was to a funny quote, or a joke I made up, I started to master the art of laughing in the storm. Once again, I can't stress the importance of having the right attitude. The right attitude is everything.

The wig shop owner showed me quite a few wigs, and I found two that I really liked. My aunt was kind enough to put down the deposit while I made sure insurance would cover both of them. One was over $3,000!

After wig shopping, I couldn't help but notice the nonstop pains in my chest. I wasn't sure what was happening, but it was starting to become a nuisance. Later that night, I drove to the hospital, but before entering the emergency room, I called up and spoke to a radiologist, telling him about my port. After a few questions, he ruled out any sort of infection. He told me that it was probably fine for me to wait until Monday to call up Dr. J's office. Because I didn't want to deal with another hospital visit, I went home and tried to relax.

Today, I learned about two things: tumor necrosis and "chemo skin." One is good, the other is evil.

I couldn't deal with my chest pains any longer. I had gone in to work in the morning but couldn't ignore the waves of pain any more. I finally told one of my bosses that I needed to leave work and go to the emergency room.

At the ER, the nurse went through all of the routine questions with me about my medical history.

"Any previous medical conditions?"

"Nope."

"Do you smoke?"

"Nope."

"Drink alcohol?"

"Nope."

"Trouble breathing?"

"Nope."

"Anything else unusual besides the chest pain?"

"Nope."

I was honestly the healthiest person on the planet. Well, you know, aside from having cancer.

I was taken into a small hospital room and was told to get into one of their cute hospital gowns that I had become very familiar with. The nurse did an EKG on me. It was normal. They drew my blood to see what they could find, and the PA, who was the nicest woman ever, explained to me that I was susceptible to blood clots in my lungs.

Holy moly! I screamed in my head.

She went on to explain that if my blood work came back normal, I most likely did not have a blood clot. If my blood work showed it was at an elevated level, which she assumed it would be, then I would need a CT scan to find out for sure if I had a blood clot. She said that because of the chemo, my blood work would most likely not come back normal.

She was wrong. After I had been waiting about an hour in the room, the PA came back and told me my blood work was normal. *Amen!*

I asked her what could have been causing the pains, and what I could do to take the pain away, so she told me she was going to call Dr. J.

When she returned, she informed me that Dr. J suspected I had tumor necrosis—meaning I had some pain in my chest area because the mass in my chest was dying off. (Die, Billy Bob, die!). After just one treatment, this was incredible news. Hallelujah! So, it turns out it was a good pain. Feeling an immense amount of relief, I went back to work and was able to get some things taken care of in the office.

Around this time of having the chest pains, I also noticed my complexion started to look absolutely horrible. No joke. I had struggled with skin problems for years, but prior to beginning chemo, I had my skin under control by taking DIM and biotin. Those two vitamins were a godsend! But now, for whatever reason, my face was rebelling. It was basically giving me the middle finger as it exploded with white and red pustules. I looked at myself in the mirror and had no idea what was going on. That's when I did some research and discovered that there is such a thing called chemo skin. Apparently, some people break out during chemo. *Great!* I thought. In less than one month, I would be a bridesmaid and seeing my boyfriend (we were in a long-distance relationship) and I'd be looking hideous. Perfect.

Let me tell you, I am not exaggerating about my skin. It was so terrible that no amount of makeup could cover it. At that point, there was nothing I could do except pray, and continue to take DIM and biotin. I also began doing some research on all-natural acne products. I found a company that prides themselves in selling facial, body, and hair products that are completely natural. I ended up purchasing toner that contained aloe vera and essential oils, as well as a Manuka honey oil. Luckily, within one week, thank the good Lord, my face went back to normal. It was a miracle.

March 9, 2016

This was the day of my second chemo treatment. I had decided since the beginning that for all my treatments, I would show up looking super-cute. I'd do my hair and makeup beautifully, and get dressed up in a cute outfit. I joked that this was called chemo chic. My theory was that if I looked good, I felt good. I wanted to be the sexiest looking cancer patient there ever was. Hey, why not? I wanted to start a new movement... the chemo chic movement. I joked that in 2017, chemo chic would be hitting the runway at a popular fashion show in New York City. Hey, it could totally happen, right? Anyway, today, I wore a pair of adorable short-heeled boots with fringe on the side, paired with leggings and a tunic. My long, blonde locks were curled at the ends, cascading down my back. I strutted into the cancer center as if I was going on a hot date. Well, I mean, I kind of was. I had a hot date with the chemo IV pole. It was our second date. Things were heating up quickly between us.

As I hung out, receiving the chemo, a beautiful woman came over to me and introduced herself. She, too, was receiving a round of chemo. We struck up a conversation, and I learned that this woman, Muriel, had been diagnosed with non-Hodgkin's lymphoma. She needed to receive three six-hour treatments.

This was Muriel's first round of chemo, and she had clearly gotten the memo about chemo chic. Her chemo chic was on fleek! She was dressed in an adorable plaid top, jeans, and super-cute flats that had little bows on them. Her hair and makeup were done perfectly, and she was decked out in all sorts of jewelry.

Muriel marked the sixth person I had met who had lymphoma. I'd had no idea it was so common. She and I spoke all throughout my treatment, just like I had with John and Pam the first time. Time flew by once again, and my dad and Muriel's husband exchanged phone numbers and said we would all keep in touch. It's amazing how God puts the right people in your path at the right time. I was so happy to have met Muriel.

When I returned home from chemo, everything took an ugly, unexpected turn. One word: nausea. Like, nausea times a million. I wanted to die. I wanted, at that very moment, to call the mob in New York and order a hit... on myself.

There are no words to accurately describe how evil nausea from chemo was. Throwing up your guts is the absolute worst. I spent the next couple of days throwing up and becoming severely dehydrated. It was so bad that I lost five pounds in one day (as terrible as this sounds, I can't complain about that part).

I was dehydrated, yet I couldn't manage to drink. I just couldn't do it. I not only had a disgusting, metallic taste in my mouth (yet another side effect) but also couldn't make myself drink anything. I had no desire to drink, and even the thought of it made me gag.

I called Dr. J's nurse to tell her what was going on, and she had Dr. J write me out another prescription for an anti-nausea pill, only this one was to be placed on the tongue and dissolved. This would be absorbed quickly and I wouldn't have to worry about throwing it up. The only problem? It tasted so bad that the taste itself almost made me throw up.

It was crazy to me how tastes and smells during chemo would make me feel nauseous and grossed-out at all times. It got to the point that certain shampoos, body washes, soaps, and other hygiene products made me nauseous at just one sniff. I had to completely restock my bathroom with all new products.

As hard as this day was, I got through it. I kept my mind focused on the good things that would be happening in the near future: I would be in Jersey in almost two weeks, surrounded by people I loved, celebrating

Lisa's wedding. It didn't get any better than that. I knew that during that time, I would be feeling much better and, because Lisa was one of the funniest people I knew, she would be making me laugh my ass off.

So another piece of advice is this: Even during rough times, always find things to look forward to in the near future. And keep reminding yourself that the pain you are in is temporary; you aren't going to feel this way forever. Soon enough, you'll be back to your old self—only you are going to be even better, stronger, and more beautiful than you were originally.

March 11, 2016

I was so severely dehydrated that I needed to go back to the cancer center to have fluids administered through an IV. Since chemo two days before, I'd barely had anything to eat. Needless to say, I was starving. The only thing I could think of was a giant blueberry muffin.

The nurse who assisted me was a doll, but she made one small mistake that I'm certain she will never make again. After a brief conversation of small talk, she looked at me and said, "And when you lose all of your hair, don't worry! It is going to grow back looking better than ever!"

I thought, *Oh, girl, you did* not *just go there.* Now, I can't speak on behalf of anyone else, but for me, the topic of hair loss was off limits. I wanted nothing more than to pretend hair loss from chemo didn't even exist. The very thought of it gave me the worst anxiety.

I felt my eyes grow wide, like a deer in headlights. My mouth began moving slower than my mind was thinking, so the only thing I was able to get out was "Well, that's not true—I mean—I think it's just going to thin. I was told it's just going to thin…" Then the waterworks came.

The nurse, God bless her, had absolutely no idea what to do. I could tell she wanted to just run away and hide. She was sweet, though, and hadn't meant any harm. She apologized and even gave me a hug.

Because the nurse from my first chemo session had told me about hair thinning, not hair loss, I was praying hard that thinning was all I would deal with. No joke, I was literally praying I would not lose my hair. There were times when I would wake up in the middle of the night and check my head because I'd had a nightmare of being bald. Yeah, I was *that* consumed by the whole hair thing.

I finished up the fluids, and the nurse released me. I had managed to calm down and tried not to think about my hair too much. I felt much better thanks to being hydrated again.

After we left the cancer center, my mom took me to a bakery. Sadly, they didn't have any blueberry muffins, but they did have scones. That was good enough. Praise the Lord, that scone was glorious.

Later that night, it started happening: hair thinning. I had just finished blow-drying my long, golden locks and happened to glance at my hairbrush. My hairbrush looked like another human's head was attached to it. I couldn't even see the bristles because they were covered in my hair.

I froze. I didn't know what to do in that moment, so I did the only thing I knew to do: freak out and cry. From that point on, brushing my hair was a traumatizing experience because a ton of hair came out each time. I knew I had to calm down, though. At this point, the only hope I had was to simply believe that my hair would thin, not fall out altogether—but the more I tried not to think about it, the more obsessed I became.

March 19, 2016

There's a saying we have all heard: "You are what you eat." What I've come to learn is this instead: "You are what you speak."

Long before my diagnosis, or even my sister's diagnosis, I began listening to a pastor who is broadcast on TV. He has written several books, and one of the things he teaches is the power of our words and how crucial it is to speak positively. In one of his books, he stresses the importance of how our words can become our reality and how we should therefore walk around saying things such as "I am healthy" and "I am blessed." That makes perfect sense if you think about it. Think of people you have met who were bitter and negative. It seems like they always have something to complain about. Have you ever noticed how their mental and physical states never changed? It's because they keep telling themselves they are sick and miserable, so they stay that way.

I strongly believe in the power of words and the power of positive thinking, so I wanted to put this to the test. Every morning, I decided to begin my day by saying to myself that I was blessed, healthy, happy, healed, and so on. I would also thank God in advance for accelerated healing, and for not losing my hair. At first, I felt kind of silly talking to myself, but I knew that for this to work, I needed to declare these things repeatedly. If you keep doing this, the good things you say soon become embedded in your mind.

Even though what you are going through is crappy, your words have the power to change things for the better. Don't get me wrong—there will be days where you just want to complain about how horrible you feel, and that is perfectly understandable. The key is to do the best you can to stay positive. Never tell yourself that you are never going to get better, or that this cancer is going to defeat you. Instead, keep saying that this cancer is temporary and that with each day that passes, you get healthier and stronger. You need to stay positive throughout this whole journey, even in the toughest times.

March 20, 2016

Today, I saw my family for dinner. I was wearing a shirt that was somewhat low-cut. As I moved my long hair away and out of my face, exposing my sternum area, my aunt immediately turned to my mom and said, "Look, the bump in her chest is gone." That's when they both proudly brought it to my attention.

Up until that point, I really hadn't noticed because I tried not to look. I hated seeing the grotesque port sticking out of my flesh, so I often tried not to look at myself naked.

As soon as my family alerted me of this great news, I had to take a look for myself. I saw for myself that Billy Bob Bump was no more. My sternum was almost completely flat and back to normal. I was in complete astonishment. Suddenly, part of me felt normal again.

RIP, Billy Bob.

Today was the day I had been dreaming about for what seemed like forever. My parents dropped me off at the airport so I could hop on my flight to Jersey. At this point, I still had hair (a lot of hair, believe it or not) on my head, which showed that the nurse from my chemo teach class had been completely wrong. I felt magnificent at knowing that I got to go back home to Jersey looking like my regular self, no wig needed.

Because I basically had no immune system thanks to the chemo robbing me of my white blood cells, I needed to wear a mask at the airport and on the plane. I felt ridiculous, but at the same time, I would never see my fellow passengers ever again, so who cared? It was much better than risking getting sick and having my trip ruined.

Here's another tip for you: Become a germaphobe. As I already mentioned, thanks to chemo, you basically don't have an immune system during this time. So, make sure you wash your hands religiously, and if your oncologist approves it, begin taking Vitamin C every day. Also, make sure you keep hand sanitizer with you at all times, especially when you are out in public. The last thing you want is to catch a cold during this time.

Later that day, when I saw Lisa, we laughed and joked like we always had. In that moment, I was normal. I forgot about everything going on in my personal life. I felt healthy and energized, too. I had brought my medications with me just in case, but I didn't need them. It was a glorious feeling.

I loved being back home in Jersey. I didn't ever want to leave.

March 25, 2016

Lisa's wedding was beautiful. Not just beautiful, but exquisite—everything, from her dress to the venue to the reception. It was all perfect. And people who didn't know me couldn't tell I was going through cancer. I think it was a mix of makeup and a positive attitude. Oh, and my hair, which got quite a few compliments, thanks to the stylist who curled it for me early in the day. I had told her to be as gentle as possible because of how fragile it was, and she had done a terrific job. It felt really good being Jen the bridesmaid and not Jen the cancer patient, and I felt incredibly grateful.

March 27, 2016

The whole hair thinning situation started to get really annoying. My hair started getting everywhere—and I mean *everywhere*. And because I was staying with my boyfriend during my trip, his condo soon turned into Jersey's very first museum of human hair, with my locks all on display. Strands of my hair were on the bed sheets, couch, floor, and bathroom. Strands even ended up in my butt crack. Luckily, I was able to laugh about it, but it started becoming an annoyance, not to mention super-embarrassing.

The good news was that aside from the hair thinning, I continued to feel completely healthy and fine during my trip. There were times when I actually forgot about what I was dealing with, because I felt so great. On that trip, everything was perfect.

When my boyfriend dropped me off at the airport, things started going south real fast. I purposely hadn't put makeup on that day because I knew I'd be crying. I cried before leaving for the airport, at the airport, and even on the plane. Not only did I not want to leave Jersey and be apart from my boyfriend and best friends, but I didn't want to go back to life in Colorado. I didn't want to go to another chemo session and go through all that discomfort and sickness again. I had felt so good during my trip and wanted that to last forever.

On the plane, I wrote myself a note to look back on once this journey was over. Here's what it said:

> One day, you will look back on this moment. This is going to be a memory soon. Just like soon the chemo will be a memory. You'll one day be able to say, "Hey, remember the time I had Hodgkin's lymphoma? Remember that time I beat cancer?"

> Right now, this seems tough; however, you are equipped for this. You are a lot stronger than you realize, so quit feeling sorry for yourself and find that strength. This is simply a season of discomfort. Going through cancer sucks, but you are going to come out of this stronger and healthier than ever before. You are going to be blessed beyond belief. The life you've always wanted is just around the corner. Don't give up, and don't you ever, ever lose your faith. Your faith is what's going to get you through to the other side. Your faith is the only thing that matters right now.

April 1, 2016

Here I was again at another fun-filled chemo session. Because this was April Fools' Day, I was waiting for Dr. J to say, "You don't have cancer! April Fools!" That didn't happen, though. Instead, as my friend Emily had come with me, the two of us spent most of the time laughing and goofing off as the poison entered my body.

Because of my prior experience with the extreme nausea, the nurse gave me a hardcore anti-nausea medication before my chemo session began. It was called Emend, and it was a godsend. The nurse assisting me today was the same one who had given me fluids the previous month and accidentally made me cry. She was a very sweet person and did her best to make me feel as comfortable as possible today.

Emily and I hung out and laughed as if we were two gals putting on a show at a comedy club. (Here's another piece of advice: Find the funniest friend you know and ask that friend to join you at chemo. Surround yourself with people who have a good sense of humor. There's nothing wrong with laughter during a chemo session!)

After chemo was over, Emily and I went to a local fast food joint for some burgers. The reason I wanted to eat a burger was because I really didn't care for burgers. I knew that if I needed to add burgers to my list of "bad foods," I wouldn't be heartbroken over it.

After we ate, I said good-bye to Emily and went back to my parents' house. Thank God I didn't get nauseous or sick. I did, however, get very tired, which was perfectly fine with me. I'd gladly take fatigue over vomiting any day! I spent the rest of the day sleeping. I dreamed of being cancer-free.

This was probably one of the roughest days for me since being diagnosed. Not only was I incredibly weak, but it was very difficult for me to concentrate at work. I was also still having a major issue with foods and my sense of taste, and I wanted nothing more than to just throw up. It was one of those days when I cried at work and then told myself, "Pull yourself together. No crying allowed. You are not weak."

I got sent home early from work because one of my bosses could sense I wasn't feeling well. He was absolutely right—I was having a majorly off day and was mentally and physically exhausted.

When I got home, I tried eating a salad but quickly realized I couldn't because it was on my list of "bad foods." I went into the bathroom to take a shower, and that's when I completely lost it. Probably for the first time, I cried without feeling guilty. For the longest time, I had told myself that if I cried, I was weak. That was a silly thing to think, and it couldn't have been further from the truth. Truth is, we are human. We have beating hearts and are created to feel emotions. We can't be stoic and emotionless, because that's not reality. We need to let our feelings out. With that in mind, I cried like a baby, and it felt really good.

Another lovely side effect of chemo is that you can become one of the most emotional people in the world. I'm not joking. I developed the talent of crying at the drop of a hat for any and every reason. At first, I just thought I was a hot mess. In reality, something about the chemo rattles all of your emotions and heightens everything. I also began feeling ultra-sensitive and irritable.

Everything started to feel… weird. I mean, there really aren't any words to describe how you feel during chemo. I simply stopped feeling like myself. Sometimes I would look at myself in the mirror and see my vacant eyes and feel completely unrecognizable. During times like those, it's important to stay focused and keep reminding yourself that you will come out of this stronger and better than ever before. The key is to not lose sight of the blessings that will be coming your way after your cancer journey is over. But to receive those blessings, you need to stay in faith and stay positive.

Whenever you have days similar to the one I had on this day, remember that it's okay to cry, and allow yourself to feel however you wish. Also remember that it's important to keep cheering yourself on. Keep that PMA, and remind yourself that you are one day closer to being healed of cancer.

April 5, 2016

For the rest of the week, I couldn't concentrate one bit. I would be at work, staring at my computer, asking myself, "What the hell am I doing?" It would take me ten minutes to write a simple e-mail. My body felt like it was shutting down, and that was starting to scare me. How was I going to be able to work if I couldn't concentrate? It felt like a mix of being really tired plus having my head in the clouds. That's when I discovered yet another side effect of chemo: fatigue. And yes, the side effects just kept coming.

Up until that moment, I had simply thought fatigue was another word for being tired. Nope. It was then that I researched fatigue and how it related to chemo, and that was when I discovered that fatigue is a much more intense version of being tired. Being tired is a few yawns, wishing you were on the couch and drinking coffee. Fatigue is when your body is worn out and no amount of coffee can help with it.

I went the rest of the week feeling fatigued and completely helpless. That resulted in lots of tears because of how useless I felt. Imagine just not feeling like yourself. Imagine going from a vibrant, energetic twenty-something-year-old to a worn-out old lady. That's how I felt. Things I had once been able to do soon became difficult to accomplish. I never once cried because I felt sorry for myself, but I would cry because of how helpless I felt.

Thankfully, by the weekend, I was back to normal… or should I say "normal"? Let's face it: During chemo, even when you feel normal, you still don't feel 100%. Things felt like they were getting better, and that's when I started regaining hope that all this crap I was dealing with was temporary. And that's what you need to keep telling yourself, because it's true. You are dealing with an illness, but that illness is not permanent. Soon, that illness is going to be a memory. A really, really crazy memory.

April 9, 2016

Today, I made the decision to cut my long locks up to my shoulders. The thinning was getting annoying, and I'd had enough of it. I was getting tired of pulling freakishly long strands of hair off my clothes, bed, and everywhere in between. I decided enough was enough and went for it, having my stylist cut it nice and short.

Originally, I was going to donate my hair to an organization that made wigs for cancer patients. The only problem was that my hair was color-treated, and they didn't accept color-treated hair. I was really sad that my hair went to waste, but I didn't have a choice.

I'm not going to lie—I loved my new 'do. Short hair is so easy to manage, and it was a really nice change for me.

If you decide not to shave your head during chemo, here's a pointer: Don't wash your hair too often. I started washing my hair once or twice a week at most. I know that sounds gross, but the more you leave your hair alone, the more of a chance you have of keeping it on your head. I also began using shampoo and conditioner made especially for hair loss. Even better, the company that made it was the same all-natural company that made the acne products I mentioned earlier.

Always be mindful of the body products you use. Try to opt for natural and organic products when possible. You don't want all those icky chemicals seeping into your pores, which will then travel to all of your organs. You want to try to keep your body as free of chemicals as possible. I mean, bad enough we need to have chemo pumped into our systems. I think that's enough poison for a lifetime.

One other hair tip: Stop blow-drying your hair or using a flat iron. Like I already mentioned, try not to do a whole lot to your hair.

If you decide to cut your hair rather than just shave it all off, embrace your new look! Get creative and play around with what makes you feel comfortable. In case you haven't noticed, short hairdos are the new trend for women, so go on and be trendy!

True friendship is when your two best friends from Jersey fly out to be with you during one of your treatments. My two best friends, Heather and Lisa, flew in so they could be with me during a chemo session. What's even sweeter is that this was Heather's birthday, and she came anyway. I bet she never in a million years thought she would ever spend her birthday at a cancer center.

Heather and Lisa's visit came at just the right time, because on that day, I realized that each treatment was harder than the previous one. Today, simply walking into the cancer center and smelling that distinct odor got me nauseous immediately.

I went through the motions of getting my vitals and weight checked, having blood work done, and then dealing with that horrible port flush, which started making me cringe and gag. Then, as I sat in the comfortable recliner waiting for my next round of poisoning to begin, I began to tear up a little.

"What's wrong, sweetie?" Heather asked.

"This is just… getting harder," I explained as I sobbed.

I sat in the chair, trying to calm myself down as one of the nurses came over to me. Today, my nurse was the nurse from the chemo teach class, the one who had told me I was going to lose my hair. She came over to me and asked how I was doing. Then, she looked at my hair, per-plexed, and said, "Your hair…?"

"I still have it!" I proudly declared. I was thrilled that she had been wrong. It felt amazing to still have my hair, and it looked super-cute now that it was short.

After the poison started pumping into my system, Heather, Lisa, and I started to think about what food we could grab afterward. This was one of the hardest decisions because it had to be a food I didn't care about, like burgers. It had to be a food that I would be okay with never wanting to think about ever again. I went through the long list of possibilities and finally decided on sandwiches.

After chemo was over, we went to a local sandwich shop. Then I slept for the rest of the day.

April 15, 2016

I attempted to go to work, hoping I would last a full day. I lasted until noon.

The nausea was under control, but it was still lingering. Although I didn't throw up this time around, I still felt like I wanted to. I just felt so gross and uncomfortable.

After I got home, I collapsed on the bed, still in my work clothes and heels, and almost fell asleep like that. Heather and Lisa woke me up so I could get into my pajamas. The rest of the day was honestly a blur. I'm pretty certain it involved lots of sleep.

April 16, 2016

Let me take this opportunity to talk to you about something else I discovered during this journey. Two words: chemo brain. If you have never heard of chemo brain (I hadn't until I began experiencing it), then let me explain it to you.

During chemo, it is common to start becoming forgetful. Your mind may feel a bit foggy. What you need to understand is that this is normal. I began noticing that my memory had gone to crap. I would forget so many different things, and sometimes it would be really hard for me to think straight. You can thank chemo for this.

Although, to my knowledge, there is really nothing you can do about this, I started to keep a pen and paper with me at all times. I would constantly write things down so I wouldn't forget them. I would also keep notes in my phone. Writing things down really helped me.

I'm not going to lie, but chemo brain became the best excuse for everything. If I accidentally forgot something, or had a "blonde moment," I would innocently shrug my shoulders and say, "Oops, sorry. I have chemo brain." No one can get mad at you for that!

I realized that I will probably use the chemo brain excuse for the rest of my life.

April 18, 2016

Heather and Lisa both left to go back home, and during this time, I began feeling so much better. I was amazed at how resilient the human body was. I always felt like absolute crap the first three days after chemo, but then, after that, I would start feeling much, much better. I would, for the most part, be able to go to work and get a ton of things done. I was able to stay on top of e-mails, deadlines, and everything in between. I felt really proud of myself for being able to go to work as I battled cancer.

At work, I felt like I was still able to act as if nothing was wrong in my personal life. I walked around the office with a smile on my face, always having a positive and upbeat attitude. I felt great when I went in to work because I enjoyed my job and being around the people I worked with. At work, I was in my "safe zone," where cancer didn't exist. At work, I was normal, or at least as normal as possible for my situation.

On this day, however, I learned that there had been a lot of talk about me in the office. It only made sense, since I was missing a ton of work. I was unsure of how to handle this. I mean, one of the reasons I hadn't made a huge announcement about my health issue was so people in the office wouldn't feel uncomfortable around me. Now I felt like if there was speculation, they would feel uncomfortable regardless. I honestly was unsure of how to deal with this appropriately, so I took a step back and made the decision to still act like nothing was wrong. More than anything, I didn't want to taint this "safe zone" I had. It was the only place I could go where I wasn't a cancer patient. I couldn't let that slip away.

April 27, 2016

Here we go again. I woke up at my parents' house and prepared for another round of chemo. Like I did all of the other times, I made sure my hair and makeup looked flawless. I picked out an outfit that was chemo chic. I put lidocaine on my port an hour prior to my chemo session. And, most importantly, I made sure I ate a good breakfast, because attempting to eat anything afterward would be incredibly difficult.

At the cancer center, I began having massive anxiety when it came to getting the routine blood work done through my port. It wasn't because of the poking or prodding, and it wasn't because of having blood drawn. Those things didn't bother me. What killed me was the saline taste that flooded my mouth when they flushed my port. I had never liked it from the beginning, but I was now at the point where every smell and taste in creation made me want to throw up.

I sat there, cringing. I had pulled out a piece of candy to suck on to help keep the saline taste at bay. I guess it was terribly obvious how miserable I was, because one of the lab techs looked at me and said, "Jennifer, you're not smiling today. What's going on?"

Part of me was sad that he noticed I wasn't wearing my usual smile. Today, though, I couldn't help it. As each second passed, I grew more and more anxious. I was almost done getting my blood drawn and I knew what was next.

"It's just… this awful taste," I explained as I violently sucked on the candy in my mouth, hoping I could extract every last bit of flavor to mask the awful saline taste. "It makes me feel so sick."

And then there it came. The taste invaded my mouth and took over my taste buds. I instantly wanted to throw up. I got incredibly nauseated. I was shaking. My palms were sweaty.

After I was dismissed from the lab section of the cancer center, I needed to go to the bathroom. Here's another crazy fact about how sensitive I was to smells: I could no longer use the hand soap in the cancer center. The evil aroma of it killed me. I had to begin bringing my own hand soap with me to chemo.

As I sat in the recliner and waited for chemo to begin, I continued to feel nauseous. I didn't know what to do with myself. I wanted to run away and hide, but knew I couldn't. I explained everything to the nurse who would be administering my chemo that day. She got Dr. J's permission to give me an extra dose of anti-nausea meds.

This extra dose, I would come to find, would make me very sleepy. Before I knew it, I was passed out in the chair. My parents were with me, both reading and checking e-mails while I slept.

Before I knew it, the day's chemo session was over. I had slept the entire time, and I was grateful that I had. I didn't want to remember those painful memories.

April 30, 2016

My intention was to walk to the bathroom and put some clean clothes on. I was feeling pretty weak, so before I reached my destination, I just needed to sit down and rest for a minute. I was at my parents' house because they always took care of me after chemo. I sat down on the floor in one of the bedrooms of their home, and across from me was a full-length mirror. I caught a glimpse of my reflection and just stared at myself for a while. I wasn't wearing makeup, yet my skin was flawless. The "chemo skin" that had once plagued me seemed to be gone for good. My eyes were tired, yet they were bright. My hair was dirty yet still intact, on my head, and clinging for dear life.

I stopped and took it all in. Then, I stared at myself dead in the eyes and said, "You're not weak. You're going to fucking conquer cancer. That's it."

There are times when, as silly as it sounds, you just need to give yourself a pep talk. You are your biggest cheerleader, and you have the power to control your thoughts. During your cancer journey, you are going to be on an emotional roller coaster. One moment, you may feel fine, and then the next, you may feel sad or upset. Both your body and mind are going through a very intense journey. Just know this: Whatever emotions you feel are perfectly okay. Simply allow yourself to feel. Make sure, though, that you are also doing what you can to stay positive. As I already mentioned, you need to keep a good attitude during this time. So my advice is to become aware of your emotions. If you need to cry, then cry. If you need to feel sad, feel sad. But the key is to then get those feelings out of your system and replace them with positive ones. Don't be afraid to stare at yourself in the mirror, like I did, and remind yourself of how strong you are.

You, my friend, are a warrior. I challenge you to make a habit of letting yourself know that every single day.

May 1, 2016

Yesterday was one of the most important days of my sister's life. Yesterday, 22-year-old Danielle graduated from college in Tulsa, Oklahoma. Now, I know that this in itself is a great achievement; however, Danielle took it to a whole other level.

As I already mentioned, Danielle was diagnosed with melanoma within five months of me being diagnosed. Her diagnosis came first. She was going about her life, working her ass off to become a nurse. All of a sudden, things came crashing down. She was in her senior year, so close to graduating, when the terrible news of her health issue came.

Danielle needed two separate surgeries to remove lymph nodes in her leg and groin area. The first surgery wasn't nearly as intense as the second. The second left her susceptible to lymphedema and also left a large scar on the back of her leg, which made her terribly self-conscious.

Both of Danielle's surgeries were performed at MD Anderson, Houston's world-renowned cancer hospital, where she was taken very good care of. After the second surgery, Danielle went back to Tulsa, where she was going to school. That was when she learned she needed to begin treatment with Yervoy. Yervoy is a treatment designed specifically for melanoma patients. Like with any medication or treatment, there were a slew of possible side effects. Unfortunately for Danielle, she was hit hard with these side effects. After just one dose of the treatment, Danielle began spending more time in the hospital than at her apartment. She had lost a ton of weight and was unable to eat because of the severe colitis that she had developed. To say Danielle was sick during this time would be a complete understatement. She literally almost lost her life.

During that entire time, I never once heard Danielle say things like "Why me?" or "Why couldn't this have happened to somebody else?" I never heard complaining from her. Instead, she made it her mission to document her journey through social media to bring awareness of skin cancer. She conducted herself with maturity and displayed an immense amount of strength. Did she feel sad? Definitely. Did she cry often? Of course. But Danielle looked to the future. She focused on all of her goals, as well as on becoming a cancer survivor. So, despite battling cancer, missing countless days of school, and being at the brink of death, Danielle still managed to graduate from nursing school with her class.

Danielle is proof that miracles still exist. She did something that happened only because of the goodness of God. I could never get through nursing school, let alone nursing school while battling cancer. Danielle did the impossible, and she did it thanks to God. Let this be a lesson to you all that even if the odds are against you, and even if something seems impossible, God can show up and make things happen that we could never make happen on our own. God is moved by our faith. If you, like Danielle, keep the right attitude and show God that you are trusting in Him to get you through a difficult time, that's when He can do the impossible. That's when He can not only heal you of cancer, like he did for Danielle, but can also make your dreams come true.

Danielle is now cancer-free and working as a nurse at one of the best hospitals in Denver.

May 11, 2016

Although today was another round of chemo, I was pretty stoked that I would be able to spend it with Muriel, as she, too, had another round today.

I'm not going to lie—today was even harder than my last round. I sat in a recliner next to Muriel as nausea plagued me. I became incredibly distraught and uncomfortable. Squirming in my chair, I secretly dealt with my feelings, hoping they would go away. I was with my mom for today's session, and Muriel was with her husband, Mike. The four of us sat near each other. I tried to engage in conversation, with the hope that the awful feelings that were eating me alive would magically disappear.

It was hard to pay attention to what anyone was saying, though, so I explained how sick I felt. I couldn't get comfortable in the chair, and I just wanted, more than anything, to throw up. I tried taking a deep breath to calm myself down. Mike then prayed over me, asking God that I would feel better.

One of the nurses got me a lemon-lime soda to drink. It sat on the table next to me, unopened. I was once again at the point where I really wanted to drink but simply couldn't.

Muriel had brought some adult coloring books with her to the session. "How about we color?" she asked. She handed me and my mom Christian-themed coloring books, with Bible verses on the pages, and a slew of neon-colored markers. I took one of the markers and began focusing my attention on coloring. To tell you the truth, it helped a lot. Taking deep breaths, focusing all my attention on the coloring book, as if I was some great artist or something, I started to feel a bit better.

About halfway through, I fell asleep. I was out cold. When I woke up, chemo was over. Muriel's session was still occurring, but I was free to go. I was extremely groggy, and as I moved in and out of consciousness, I said good-bye to Muriel and Mike. When I walked out to the parking lot with my mom, I was almost convinced I was going to get sick. I didn't, though. Instead, I passed out in the car as we drove back to my parents' house.

My mom kept the coloring pages that she and I had worked on. She proudly displayed them in the kitchen, kind of like when your 6-year-old child makes artwork with macaroni. This time, though, it was her 28-year-old daughter who had created the artwork without puking all over it. That's a fair accomplishment, I'd say.

I was unable to look at those coloring pages without feeling sick.

May 13, 2016

Here is a fact: Your mind is going to want to mess with you from time to time. It can happen at any moment, too, like when you are trying to go to sleep at night, or when you have some alone time during the day. When you least expect it, negative thoughts are going to invade your mind and try to steal your hope and faith. Those thoughts may take you back to your last chemo session to remind you of the horror you endured. Or they might whisper lies to you, saying, "You'll never get better. That PET scan isn't going to come back clear." What you need to do is be prepared.

Think back to an extremely pleasant memory you have. Maybe it involves your significant other or best friend. Or think about one of the goals that you want to achieve after you are done with chemo. Keep this memory or goal locked away and on guard. The next time any negative thoughts creep up on you, say, "No thanks!" and knock them out with your pleasant memory or goal, and simply begin focusing on that memory or goal instead.

As I already mentioned, you need to stay strong mentally. I wholeheartedly believe that if you have the right attitude, you will get through even the most difficult times. So the next time your mind wants to wander in the wrong direction, don't let it. Immediately bring it back to focus on pleasant thoughts. Remember, you control your thoughts. Sometimes we can't help but let our thoughts mess with us; that is bound to happen. The key is to not dwell on those things. We have the power to flip the switch and bring our attention to something positive.

Remember: You are in control of you. You have the power to control your attitude and your thoughts. Even though it can be easier said than done, stay strong. You're almost at the finish line.

May 16, 2016

Here's a riddle for you: What is worse than recovering from a round of chemo while also PMS-ing?

The answer: Nothing. There is nothing worse than dealing with the aftermath of chemo while also dealing with the joys of womanhood. Seriously. *Nothing*.

I'm not going to lie—this day was rough. And it was Monday, no less. Everything started at 3 a.m., when I woke up and couldn't fall back to sleep. Every time I tossed and turned, all I felt was the loose hairs on my pillowcase clinging to my face and refusing to get off. That was a common thing these days. Each morning, I would wake up and see hair that had once been on my head lying on my pillowcase. And each morning, I would try very hard not to have a nervous breakdown.

After tossing and turning, peeling hairs off my face, and scrutinizing just how many strands I had lost overnight, I decided to begin my day.

This was the first day since my chemo treatment on Wednesday that I put makeup on. I did my usual makeup routine, and after I was done, I couldn't help but feel… *strange.* Usually, after that last swipe of mascara, I felt put together and ready to take on the world. Not today, though. I couldn't pinpoint it right away, but I just didn't feel like myself. And as I began to scrutinize my appearance, I didn't recognize myself, either. My hair was a hot mess, first of all. Although I still had hair on my head— thank God—it had thinned so badly that you could almost see my scalp on the top of my head, where I part my hair. I needed to start parting it differently and wear headbands to cover up the thinning.

My eyebrows had also thinned a lot, which isn't really a complaint, just an observation. I hadn't had to pluck my eyebrows since… I couldn't even remember. My eyelashes were also extremely sparse. Once upon a time, they had been long and thick. Now they were barely there. I felt like suddenly, I changed. I just didn't feel like myself.

In that moment of Monday misery, I started to obsess over my appearance. I started criticizing how awful my hair looked. Because I couldn't flat-iron it or style it that much, I had begun to let it air dry. The less I did to it, the better. I didn't want to do anything that would make it fall out. Anyway, after a brief pity party, something deep down inside of me told me to knock it off. I then thought, *Shame on me. Some people don't even have hair thanks to chemo. I kept my hair, and I have the audacity to complain?* I felt awful. I was blessed in so many ways, and that was what had helped me make it this far. Even though my appearance was slightly different, I still looked fine. I decided in that moment to stop obsessing about how I looked. Easier said than done, I know, but eventually, hair grows back. Eyelashes grow back. Everything would soon go back to normal.

Here's probably one of the worst things, in my opinion, about going through chemo: You begin associating everything with chemo. I kid you not. You may associate foods, drinks, smells, items… the list goes on. For example, on that morning, before I left for work, I went to grab something out of my purse. Keep in mind that this was the same purse I used every day, including when I went to chemo. Because I had been cooped up in the house since my last round, I had not used my purse since then. I reached for something in my purse and was instantly brought back to my last chemo session. My purse actually smelled like the cancer center. And because I was also PMS-ing and super-emotional, I started bawling immediately. I was instantly brought back to terrible memories of nausea and sickness. Needless to say, this made me realize that I had a great excuse to go out and buy a new purse.

On the drive to work, I started thinking of how I didn't want to ever go back to the cancer center. Once again, because I felt like everything was hitting me all at once, I started bawling in my car. And then I started crying because I didn't want to cry. And then I started crying on top of that because I was pissed that I had just ruined all my makeup.

During the day, I ran into the bathroom a couple of times because I was crying so hard. Thankfully, no one I worked with witnessed this. I was just super-emotional and there was no way to stop it.

Here's the thing: Even though this was a less-than-ideal kind of day, I got through it, and I felt proud of myself for getting through it. Sure, it wasn't a second thought to some people to make it through the day, but it meant everything to me because it was a small achievement. Days like this specific one are inevitable. Because you're going to be ultra-sensitive and irritable thanks to chemo, you will have some sucky days. That's just how it is. Just keep telling yourself that you are going to make it through.

When things start to get overwhelming, take five minutes to take a short walk or go somewhere private. Try to quiet your mind and silence any negative thoughts. Just know that you will make it through, and that tomorrow will be a better day.

May 21, 2016

I had received the news that my insurance didn't cover wigs. My aunt had already made the deposit, but learning that the wigs would be full price was upsetting to me. My aunt generously bought one of the wigs for me, despite having to pay the full price. I was so grateful for this.

The wig was beautiful and looked natural. I named her Sonia. Sonia was blonde, had some layers, and looked similar to my old hair. Sonia was fierce and fabulous.

This was the first day I wore Sonia in public. I knew it would take some time to get used to wearing her. For example, as I strutted around the mall, even though I felt great, I noticed I couldn't really look people in the eye. I thought maybe in the back of my mind, I feared people would know I was wearing a wig. I knew it would take some time to get used to, but I also knew it was silly for me to feel self-conscious. I'm pretty sure no one could tell, and even if they could, who cared? They were complete strangers I would never see again.

During one of my errands, I popped into the makeup store because I needed an eyebrow pencil. Because my eyebrows had thinned, as I have already mentioned, I wanted an eyebrow pencil to darken them up a little. I had never needed to use one before, so I was hoping one of the makeup artists there could help me and show me what the heck to do.

When one of the makeup artists asked if I needed anything, I said, "Yes. I need eyebrows."

She and I started chatting, and before I knew it, she had given me an entire makeover with all new makeup. Keep in mind, I'd been using the same makeup for years, and it was the mineral kind that didn't really give full coverage.

After the makeup artist was done, she told me to look in the mirror. I was amazed at how great I looked. Not only was my skin radiant, but I had eyebrows again!

I walked out of the store with $66 worth of new makeup.

What I learned was that even though our appearances can change during chemo, that shouldn't stop us from looking or feeling our best. Don't be afraid of change. Embrace it. And don't be afraid to play around with your look while you're going through chemo. Even if you have lost your eyelashes and eyebrows, you can still buy some fake eyelashes to wear, and you can pencil your eyebrows in. I mean, even people who still have their eyelashes and eyebrows do that! Think of celebrities—they spend an insane amount of money on hair extensions, wigs, fake eyelashes, makeup, etc. Why can't we do that too and splurge on ourselves? Don't be afraid to be a little elaborate and reinvent your look. It will give you the boost of confidence that you need during this time.

If you don't feel comfortable spending a lot of money on makeup, do some research on certain cancer organizations that give free makeup classes for cancer patients. They not only teach you to do your makeup but also give you a big bag full of free makeup from well-known brands. It doesn't get any better than that!

I woke up on this morning to a pounding heart as I remembered what day it was—my seventh chemo treatment. I lay there in bed and tried to take deep breaths to calm myself. It didn't work. I felt like a toddler whose mother had just told her that she was going to the doctor for a shot. I kept repeating, in my little toddler voice, "I don't want to go, I don't want to go." I threw a tantrum in my head.

I chose my chemo chic outfit, applied my new makeup immaculately, and kept trying to stay calm. I felt like a hypocrite in that moment because though I was trusting in God, I was still anxious about the upcoming treatment.

At the cancer center, I waited in the doctor's office to meet with Dr. J. As I waited to meet with him, I suddenly felt really sick. I ran into the bathroom and threw up my guts. Lovely. Nausea after chemo is normal, but *before*? I felt so sick that I wished I could run out of the cancer center right then and there.

I met with one of the nurses before meeting with Dr. J and explained what had just happened. She had then told Dr. J, and when he walked in, asking what was going on, I said, "I was just so excited to see you that I threw up."

Then I learned that what I had just experienced was called anticipatory nausea. Dr. J told me that for the next time, I should take my anti-nausea/anti-anxiety pill the night before chemo, as well as in the morning before coming to the cancer center. They would also be administering that same drug to me today, through the IV.

For this day's session, both my sister and Emily accompanied me. We sat down in the chemo room and waited for things to begin. Emily, as I already mentioned, was one of the funniest people I knew. She brought along a picture book of hairstyles—not just any hairstyles, but the really bad ones from all different eras. It gave us a really good laugh.

I actually fell asleep really fast, thanks to the meds the nurse gave me. Everything after that was a blur. At one point, I woke up briefly and saw Emily "reading" her hair book. I then passed out once again right away.

Later that night, I realized that my next chemo treatment would be my eighth. I remembered that Dr. J had said I would need anywhere from four to six cycles, or eight to twelve individual rounds. That's when my heart danced because I knew that my next round would be my last. That would be it. I was confident that I was already healed of cancer. There was simply no way I would need any more chemo after my eighth treatment.

May 28, 2016

Life threw a curveball at me today. Dealing with cancer in itself is obviously hard enough, but dealing with cancer while someone you love walks out of your life? Well, that, my friends, is completely devastating.

On this day, my boyfriend decided that he wanted to break up with me. He had been in my life for eight years, and I had grown to love him so much that my heart hurt. As we spoke on the phone—remember, we had a long-distance relationship—he laid the news on me very matter-of-factly, letting me know that he didn't see a future with me. There was no emotion in his voice. He had not one ounce of sympathy. I held it together on the phone and thanked him for being honest.

I was so blindsided that I had no idea what else to say. Here I was, almost finished with chemo, almost getting ready to begin the next chapter of my life, and suddenly, someone I had never expected would hurt me went and did something like that. Now what? What was going to happen next?

The truth is, whether during your cancer journey or not, you are going to have people walk out of your life for one reason or another. Don't try to figure it out—just like you shouldn't try to figure out why you got cancer. It's okay to not have all the answers. The only thing that matters is that God has the answers. He knows what is best for us, and the key is to simply trust Him no matter what.

I spent the rest of my day in tears, trying to mourn the loss of my relationship. In that moment of complete devastation, something rose up inside of me. There was that little voice that screamed out, "You are strong. You are going to get through this." I knew that God had closed the door on my relationship because that relationship wasn't what was best for me. It didn't matter that I didn't know that specific reason; what mattered was that God knew that reason. I realized in that moment that I needed to keep trusting God and passing these tests. I wanted to make Him proud of me, and I wanted Him to know that whatever came my way in life, I could handle with grace and maturity.

When someone you love walks out of your life, especially if that person chooses to walk out on you as you are battling cancer, let them go. People who turn their backs on you as you are in the middle of battling an illness don't deserve your tears, energy, or time. You need to go back to your mental happy place and focus on the goals or pleasant memories that bring you joy. Take time to heal from the loss, but also realize that you cannot allow that person to hinder the healing of your body. Even though dealing with the pain someone has left you with is going to hurt, try to reason with yourself. Keep reminding yourself that you can't let anything get in the way of your body healing from cancer. Remember that *you* are your number-one priority. Know your self-worth, and never settle for anything less than you deserve. Soon, you will be a cancer survivor, not a cancer patient, and you deserve to be treated with all the love and respect in the world.

May 30, 2016

This was Memorial Day, so I had the day off work. I went to visit my friend Blythe, who was currently battling breast cancer. I know God put her in my life for a reason, and I am beyond happy that He did. We both encouraged one another almost daily, and I always enjoyed seeing her because of her kind and genuine nature.

After visiting her, I went to my parents' house for a barbecue. They invited family over, along with a couple of our family friends. I wanted to look really nice, so I got decked out and put Sonia on. Keep in mind that although I still did have my hair, it was thin—thinner than thin. Like, there were no words to describe how thin. I was balding on the top of my head, and it was getting worse by the day.

This would be the third time I had worn Sonia, and I was still getting used to wearing a wig. I still felt a little self-conscious at first, but because Sonia was so natural-looking, it was an easy adjustment.

The barbecue was fun, and we all had a nice time. While we were all hanging out outside, it suddenly got really windy. Poor Sonia! I feared that she would blow away, so I excused myself to go inside for a bit. Inside, I went into one of the bedrooms to find a mirror so I could fix my makeup and have some alone time. It was during this time that I just lost it. I don't know exactly what triggered this, but I felt incredibly over-whelmed at the moment. There I was, staring at myself in the mirror, feeling unrecognizable in a wig. I just looked at myself as tears poured out of my vacant eyes.

I began beating a dead horse, going through all of the things that saddened me about my boyfriend breaking up with me. My boyfriend turned his back on me while I was going through cancer, and he will never know exactly what I went through, because he wasn't there for me. Sure, we texted often and occasionally spoke on the phone, but he had never physically been with me during my most difficult times and would therefore never know the pain I felt to see myself in a wig at first, or how many times I would break down because the feeling of his abandonment would consume me. He would never know how terrible I felt as I combed my hair and chunks would fall out, leaving me feeling more and more anxious by the second. He would never know the discomfort of chemo. He would never know how badly he had broken my heart.

I sat on the floor as all of these thoughts raced through my head. I knew I needed a good cry in order to heal. More importantly, though, I knew that this sadness was temporary.

I wiped my eyes and fixed my makeup. Then I kept reminding myself that I was going to not only get through this rough patch but also come out of it stronger and better than ever—and, more importantly, that the reason for this breakup was that God was saying no. He could see the big picture and knew what was in store for me, and for one reason or another, my boyfriend didn't belong in that picture. So, at the conclusion of my pity party, I simply thought, *Thank you, God, for having my back once again.*

With that, I walked back into the party, ate some dessert, and carried on as if no meltdown had ever occurred.

June 4, 2016

Over the course of this journey, I had many people tell me that I was handling the ordeal extremely well, that I was really mature, and that I had a positive attitude. Those compliments meant the world to me, and it made me feel good to know that people could see my light shining through, even during this dark time. It has made me realize that I was able to get through anything and everything that came my way in life. It just goes to show that I was even able to deal with getting my heart broken from someone I truly trusted.

It had been exactly one week since my ex-boyfriend had broken up with me. I felt like I had healed in this short time. Monday, two days before this, had been the last time I had cried over the breakup. On Wednesday morning, I woke up and instantly felt renewed. As I got ready for work that morning, I noticed that I had a little more pep in my step than I had the past couple of days. The sun was shining brightly, and I felt as if everything was completely fine. I felt free.

We have all heard the saying "When one door closes, another one opens." God had not only closed the door on my relationship with my ex-boyfriend but had slammed it shut, locked it, and thrown away the key. I knew deep inside that soon, another door would open and behind that door would be my future husband, who would be everything I could ever hope and dream of. I knew it was going to happen when it was meant to, and that it would be worth the wait.

June 7, 2016

On the night of June 6, there was a severe thunderstorm in my area. The sky was pitch-black, but it occasionally lit up from lightning. Thunder rumbled angrily, and hail violently crashed down on my windshield as I drove home from work. I couldn't remember the last time I had witnessed such a crazy storm. As I got closer to my apartment, I noticed flooding in some areas. Everything around me was dark and miserable.

This morning, however, I woke up to sunshine. Birds were chirping. The sky was baby blue. The ground was dry. The grass was greener than green, and the squirrels and bunnies that roam my apartment parking lot were playing. By the looks of it, you could never tell that such a storm had occurred the night before. Everything was back to normal, and there were no signs of rain or hail from the previous night.

Here's my point: The storms in our lives aren't permanent. Although we may have some thunder and hail going on around us, it isn't forever. When you start to experience a thunderstorm, grab your umbrella, but understand that it isn't going to rain forever. Soon, when you are declared cancer-free, the sun is going to come out, and it will shine more brightly than you ever thought possible. There's going to be a huge rainbow above you, blinding you with its brightness and beauty. Don't give up hope! Keep on fighting, and before you know it, the storm is going to be over.

My last treatment. *My. Last. Treatment.* I kept repeating it over and over in my head. I kept declaring to God that this was it. In two weeks, I was scheduled to have a PET scan, and I felt strongly that the scan would come back and show no evidence of cancer lurking in my body. My faith has been unshakeable this entire time, and I knew that this day, June 8, 2016, would be the last time I ever received chemo.

To help with my anxiety, I took my anti-anxiety pill the night before treatment and again on the morning of. Here's the crazy thing: I can't remember what happened next. Thank God for all the meds that got me all doped up! I remember bits and pieces of the day's treatment. I remember meeting with Dr. J briefly, and telling him that I was already completely healed and that my PET scan was going to be normal. I remember watching him cross his fingers, wanting to agree with me but knowing he couldn't until we received the actual results. I remember Muriel surprising me during chemo, giving me a gift to celebrate my last treatment. "What a sweet surprise," I think I may have said in and out of consciousness. After that, however, I don't remember a thing. I slept during most of my treatment, and I honestly don't even remember leaving the cancer center. I was out cold for the rest of the day after getting to my parents' house after treatment.

Oh, and I do remember briefly waking up from my deep slumber, bawling my eyes out. I remember hugging my dad as I cried hard. I don't know exactly why I was crying. I think it was a combination of feeling overwhelmed that this cancer journey was almost over and of feeling sad that my ex-boyfriend wasn't there for me to see me through it.

As I already mentioned, chemo can make you incredibly emotional, so if you begin crying and you're not exactly sure why, it's okay. There's nothing wrong with you, I promise.

After Cry Fest 2016, I went back to sleep. I woke up the next morning not knowing what had hit me.

June 9, 2016

This day marked exactly four months since I had been diagnosed with Hodgkin's lymphoma. In four short months, so many things had happened: so many changes in my body, so many lessons learned, so many tears cried, so many prayers answered, so many blessings received. The past four months had been a whirlwind of craziness enveloping me.

I found myself trying to process this whole journey. What I had been through in four months, at the age of 28, felt crazy to me. And for my 22-year-old sister, who had battled and conquered melanoma, even crazier. I'd been having a hard time getting my words together to accurately articulate how I was feeling, but it was really hard to do.

Think about it: Two perfectly happy and healthy sisters in their twenties were going about their lives when suddenly, within five months of each other, they were both diagnosed with cancer. You can't make this stuff up. It would have been so easy to get upset, feel defeated, and question God. It would have been normal to try to figure out why these things had happened, and to stop believing in God because, you know, why would God allow this to happen to His children?

Just the opposite happened to me, however. My faith got stronger each and every day. Since Day 1, I never questioned God. I never tried to figure out how I had gotten lymphoma. I never once got angry about my situation. Instead, I prayed relentlessly and began changing my life around. Although I had been a believer my whole life, this cancer journey got me much closer to God. I know that for whatever reason, I was meant to go through this.

Genesis 50:20 states, "As for you, you meant evil against me, but God meant it for good." Even though we can't make sense of why we had to go through cancer, we need to stay in faith, knowing that God is going to use this for our good. Since Day 1, I have been excited about using my cancer journey to help others going through cancer. I wasn't going to waste my pain. I wasn't going to go through this journey and then, when it was over, go back to my normal life and continue living for myself. No, that's not the plan. The plan is to let God direct my steps, showing me how I could help cancer patients who feel scared and hopeless. The question isn't "What do I get out of this?" but rather "What could I give from this?"

Throughout this journey, I have felt unstoppable and unbreakable. To be honest, I think another side effect of chemo is a giant boost of confidence. Like, if you could make it through cancer, you could make it through anything and everything else that comes your way. It feels like you have the world in the palm of your hands.

What the enemy wants to use to harm you, God will turn around and use for your good. The key, though, is to completely trust God. You need to wholeheartedly believe in your healing. In Mark 11:23, Jesus says, "Truly I say to you, whoever says to this mountain, 'Be taken up and thrown into the sea,' and does not doubt in his heart, but believes that what he says will come to pass, it will be done for him." God is moved by our faith. When we boldly declare that we are going to be healed of cancer, that gets His attention. That lets Him know that we are serious about our faith. That's when things start happening that we could never make happen on our own. Wake up every morning and thank God that very soon, you will be declared cancer-free.

June 12, 2016

I have already mentioned this, but when you are going through chemo, foods can become the enemy. I can safely say that about 80 percent of all foods began to disgust me. Foods I once loved, I now couldn't even think about. It had gotten to the point where even watching fast food commercials on TV disgusted me. Whenever one came on, I needed to either change the channel or close my eyes. Otherwise, it would set me off. I would begin crying at just the sight of those disgusting foods.

With that said, grocery shopping throughout this journey was one of the biggest pains ever. Before cancer, I got in and out of grocery stores at lightning speeds. I'd know exactly what I needed and would never waste any time while shopping. I'd grab what I needed and head to the checkout. I was on a mission, and no one could stop me.

That completely changed during chemo, however. I could no longer make a thorough grocery list because I really didn't like many foods. Even the foods I kind of did like, I might not crave or want to eat right away, so now when I went grocery shopping, I needed to go up every single aisle and look at every single type of food and ask myself, "Can I eat this without wanting to throw up?" Another thing that killed me was the fact that the health nut in me tried hard to eat somewhat healthily, even though it felt nearly impossible most of the time. This was usually my internal monologue when grocery shopping:

Can't get this food—it has to be microwaved. Microwaves are bad for you. Can't get this food—it has artificial dyes in it. Artificial dyes are bad for you. Can't get this food—it has too much sugar. Sugar feeds cancer cells. Can't get this food—it's not organic. Non-organic food contains pesticides. Can't get this food—it's raw. Raw foods may cause bacteria. Can't get this food—it comes in a BPA-lined can. BPA causes cancer. Can't get this food—it reminds me of chemo. Can't get this food—the smell of it makes me want to throw up.

The struggle was real, my friends. So after getting frustrated with food, walking up and down the aisles with tears in my eyes, I would grab anything that sounded decent, no matter how unhealthy it was. Sometimes I'd walk out of the grocery store with a frozen pizza and pint of ice cream. Other times, I'd be healthier and get some organic vegetables and fish.

My advice is to do the best you can when it comes to eating. Many people usually don't have an appetite during chemo. I, however, would sometimes get so hungry a few days after chemo that I would eat like a woman who was pregnant with triplets. The problem was trying to find foods that I could tolerate. Once you figure that part out, however, try to get as much down as you can. You need to eat to stay strengthened, so just do the best you can.

June 15, 2016

Oh, girl, what on God's green earth happened to you? I questioned as I looked at myself in the mirror. I had just gotten home from work and taken my headband off, exposing my sad little balding head. I don't even know how to describe what I saw. There were two patches on either side of my head where my hairline had been that were now completely bald. My scalp on top was visible, with very few strands of hair sitting on it, waiting to fall out at any given moment. When I wore a headband, it looked fine, except I realized that I also had a bald spot on the back of my head that the headband obviously didn't cover.

My first reaction after really studying this sight was to cry, so I did. And then I kind of got over it. First of all, I was in no position to complain about my appearance or hair situation, because I still had hair. It wasn't much, but it was still there, and I was still able to manipulate my look with the use of headbands. Second, because I felt so strongly in my heart that June 8 had been my last chemo treatment ever, I knew that soon, my hair would begin growing back. I would only need to endure a few more months of baldness, so I wasn't going to complain or feel sorry for myself. Further, I reminded myself in that moment, even though I didn't feel as beautiful as I used to, God still thought I was beautiful. Once you realize that the God of the universe approves of you and loves you regardless of how you look, nothing else seems to matter.

I understand that dealing with your appearance changing is very difficult, but know in your heart that this is a temporary change. Even if you feel ugly or "less than," know that you are God's child and He thinks you are amazing. And at the end of the day, the only opinion that matters is God's.

The next day, June 20, I was going to have my PET scan. That would determine how this cancer journey was going. At this point, I had done everything I could possibly do. I had prayed, stayed faithful, and declared my health and happiness every day. Now, the only thing left to do was believe. I knew I couldn't worry about my PET scan results. I knew in my heart that I was already healed. I knew that June 8 had been my last chemo treatment. I felt so strongly and had such an unshakeable faith that nothing was going to persuade me to think otherwise. I knew this entire time that God was in control, and that God was going to finish what He had started. He wasn't going to just leave me hanging toward the end of this journey.

I understand that going through cancer is rough. A lot of emotions are involved, and you really do learn a lot. And just when you think you have reached the finish line, you need to get the PET scan done to determine your health status. I get that it's nerve-wracking. What I have learned, though, is that you can't let fear take over your thoughts. You can either stay positive, telling yourself that your PET scan results are going to be fine, or stay awake at night, going through all the reasons you think your results aren't going to come back okay. Here's the key: Don't let your mind wander. Don't convince yourself that you still have cancer. This is why I believe that the daily declarations are crucial. If you wake up every morning and declare that you are healthy, happy, cancer-free, and strong, you are going to embed those positive thoughts in your mind. That is going to create the right mental state for you, and those positive words are going to take root. In contrast, if you go around saying that you are sick and weak—well, you are going to convince yourself that you aren't going to get better. Your mind is a very powerful thing. Use it wisely.

Upon waking up this morning, I didn't feel too nervous. I wasn't allowed to eat or drink prior to my PET scan, so I did my makeup and headed out the door. In the car, I still didn't feel nervous. I kept telling myself that I was going to be just fine. I thought of the people I knew who had recently received good PET scan results, like Muriel, so I thought, *Hey, if they can receive good reports, I can too!*

When I got to the hospital, the nurse took me back into a small room. I allowed him to have his way with my arm and poke and prod it with a needle. I was beyond thrilled that for my PET scan, they wouldn't need to access my port at all.

The nurse then gave me instructions. He had a little timer ticking away. When the timer went off in roughly a half hour, I needed to drink a full glass of water. Shortly after, the PET scan would begin.

The nurse dimmed the lights, and I hung out in a recliner in the small room, feeling relaxed and free from any anxieties whatsoever. To continue the good vibes, I spent this time watching a sermon from my favorite pastor on my smartphone. He was speaking about fear vs. faith. It was exactly what I needed to hear. We have the choice of living fearfully or faithfully. He spoke of how we also need to be mindful of not using our faith in the wrong way. Sometimes, we tend to have faith that bad things are going to happen to us. For example, people who believe they are going to remain sick forever convince themselves that they will never get better. If you think this way, you need to stop that kind of thinking right now. Be careful about what things you put into your mind. Believe that you *are* going to get better and that your cancer is temporary.

I had just begun to doze off in the dim room when the timer suddenly screamed at me, waking me up. I chugged the glass of water, every last drop. Finally, the nurse came to get me and took me into the main room where the PET scan would be performed. I lay down on a narrow little bed and was told to keep still. The bed began to move me back and forth through the machine.

Just as I had during the first PET scan, I kept my eyes closed the whole time to prevent me from getting claustrophobic. As the scan occurred, I kept repeating in my mind that I was cancer-free and that this scan was going to come back just fine. I recited Bible verses in my head, specifically Mark 9:23 ("All things are possible for one who believes") and Mark 5:36 ("Do not fear, only believe"). Those words were spoken by Jesus Himself, so they comforted me, like a warm blanket wrapped around me.

The PET scan, believe it or not, went much faster than I had expected. Before I knew it, I was getting off the narrow little bed and leaving the cancer center. I would be meeting with Dr. J in two days to go over my results. I felt at peace.

After my PET scan, I headed to work. I forgot about anything cancer-related. Thankfully, I was able to concentrate on getting things done in the office. My day flew by, and before I knew it, I was driving home from work. To my surprise, on the drive home, I received a phone call from Dr. J's nurse. It wasn't just *a* phone call, it was *the* phone call. I hadn't been expecting anyone to call me prior to my appointment in two days, so I was a little shocked.

"Your scan looks good," the nurse told me. "You don't need any more chemo."

As I heard those beautiful words, I almost crashed my car. Those were the words I had been praying for. The message was music to my ears. It was impossible to describe my state of mind after I heard those words. It was almost as if someone had told me I had just won the lottery. Actually, it was better than that. *No more chemo.* That was what I had declared all along, and it had finally just been confirmed!

"Wait," I told the nurse, "I just want to make sure I heard you correctly. No more chemo?"

"No more chemo!" she declared.

I was overjoyed.

The nurse then told me that, as a precaution, it was "strongly recommended" that I begin radiation treatment to make absolutely sure that all the cancer cells had been killed.

I needed to let all of this sink in, and luckily, I knew that I would receive more information in two days. Then, the nurse told me that two spots had shown up in my lungs. They were symmetrical, in both of my lungs. Dr. J believed this was a benign infection and didn't seem too concerned about it.

I couldn't be concerned, either, because in that moment, I could celebrate being healed of cancer.

When I got home, I called the people I was closest with: my parents, sister, best friends, aunts, and grandparents. Then, after informing my support system that I was healed of cancer, I completely broke down. I sat quietly in my apartment and thanked God over and over again. How do you even begin to thank God for healing you of cancer? I felt like my words were so meager. The God of the universe had healed me of cancer. He had heard every prayer that my support system and I had prayed.

My heart was filled with so much joy that I couldn't even think straight.

What I have been saying all along about positive thinking, faith, and daily declarations is true. I am proof that if you have the right attitude, stay faithful, and declare every single day that you are healthy and strong, God is going to heal you and bless you. God wants to do amazing things for us, but sometimes we don't believe that. Or sometimes we don't believe we are worthy. We think that because we have made mistakes in our lives, God won't want to help us out. The truth is, God loves us more than we can imagine. We are human, and yes, we are going to screw up. This doesn't stop God from loving us and wanting to take care of us, though.

I strongly believe that if we live every day trying to be our best, trying to please God and be good people, He will honor us. I believe that in life, we are given these small tests that we need to pass. For example, I wholeheartedly believe that when my ex-boyfriend walked out of my life, that was a test. I knew in my heart of hearts that God wanted to see how I would react if He removed someone I loved from my life. When I really think about it, I believe I passed that test with flying colors. I believe God was extremely proud of me not only for letting my ex-boyfriend go without putting up a fight but also for telling Him that I trusted Him and the things He was doing for me. And I was extremely proud of myself for passing the small tests I had been given, because they made me realize that God is always in complete control of everything.

Here's some food for thought: I have a really wonderful relationship with my dad. We have a very close and special bond. When I was little, I was a little bit of a monster child. Sometimes my dad and I would get into verbal fights, and there were times when I got off course for a little while. My dad loves me so much that even though I didn't always do the right thing, all I needed to do was tell him I was sorry, and in a flash, everything would go back to normal. I was instantly forgiven and we would carry on as if nothing had happened. Further, I knew—and still know—that if I ever needed anything, my dad would give it to me in a heartbeat because he loves me so much.

Matthew 7: 9–11 states, "Or which one of you, if his son asks him for bread, will give him a stone? Or if he asks for a fish, will give him a serpent? If you then, who are evil, know how to give good gifts to your children, how much more will your Father who is in heaven give good things to those who ask him!" This verse just goes to show that if our parents love us and want to help us when we need them, God loves us a trillion times more—more than we could imagine—and He wants to bless us. But I believe the key is what's stated in that last sentence: "to those who ask him."

So, don't be afraid to be bold. Don't be afraid to ask God to heal you of cancer. Stay in faith, and know that God loves you very much and wants to bless you. Miracles still happen, and the fact that I had such an accelerated healing and no longer needed to get chemo is proof that prayer and faith are more powerful than any treatment or medication out there.

It is impossible to describe how I had felt for the past couple of days. I could tell you that I felt happy and relieved, but those are complete understatements. I felt like I had the world in the palm of my hand. I had been healed of cancer. No more chemo. Thank you, God!

I bounced around my apartment, singing and dancing like a crazy person as I got ready to meet with Dr. J. Smiling from ear to ear, I felt unstoppable. I couldn't stop saying it: *God healed me of cancer.*

Even though I was done with chemo, I absolutely loathed being in the cancer center that day. As soon as the vestibule doors opened, *that smell* punched me in the face. I can't even describe the smell. It's just the smell of chemo. It's the smell I associate with those horrible memories of sitting in the chair, receiving poison, and feeling like hell afterward. It's *the* smell. The. Worst. Smell.

I sat in the waiting area with my parents and sister. I had joked this entire time and called them all my assistants whenever they came to the cancer center with me. Sometimes the nurses or other patients would ask me who I was there with that day. "I brought my assistant, Danielle," I would joke. Or "I have my whole team of assistants with me today." The truth is, I couldn't ask for better people to assist me during this time. I had the most wonderful family. They did an amazing job helping me out, waiting on me hand and foot after chemo, ensuring that I was as comfortable as humanly possible. I felt beyond blessed.

After the routine blood work, my assistants and I met with Dr. J. He walked in, shook our hands, and immediately declared, "The scan looks good, no need for any more chemo."

I would never get tired of hearing such beautiful words!

Dr. J checked my breathing and ruled out pneumonia. He said that the spots on my lungs were most likely a benign infection but he would monitor them. He asked if I had any shortness of breath or a persistent cough. When I told him no, he said he felt confident that there was nothing seriously wrong.

Then I learned a little bit more about the next step: radiation. Because cancer cells can be so tiny, radiation would make absolutely sure that every last cell had been destroyed. Dr. J figured I would need about a month of radiation, which would occur every day except for weekends. I was instructed to meet with a radiation doctor to get more specific information.

After the meeting, I made two new appointments: one to meet with the radiation doctor and the other to have a follow-up meeting with Dr. J. I was one step closer to being completely done with treatment and was close to officially beginning a new chapter of my life. The chapter I was currently in was filled with toxic things, like cancer and a boy who walked out on me when I needed him the most. The next chapter, however, was going to be filled with nothing but love, good health, and blessings.

June 23, 2016

This was the day of my meeting with the radiation doctor. The radiation department was in the same cancer center that I had been going to. As I walked into the cancer center, *that smell*, like always, punched me in the face, instantly making me want to throw up. I sat in the waiting area and tried to keep my mind distracted, not thinking of the smell.

Before my aunt had bought me Sonia, I had found out that a department inside the cancer center gave free wigs to cancer patients. Out of pure desperation, I had gone to check them out, to be on the safe side. I had been there a while back and picked up a wig that I named Donna. Donna was actually pretty hideous, and I never wore her, but like I said, this was out of pure desperation.

Anyway, while I was waiting to be called back to meet with the radiation doctor, I was able to return Donna. "I don't need her," I proudly declared. "I'm done with chemo." The two women working in the department were very sweet. They looked at me a bit confused, though. I was currently wearing a thick pink headband, with my little strands of hair coming out on the sides.

"That's great! Did you use the cold cap?" one of them asked me.

"Nope! I just prayed a lot!" I responded.

A really sweet nurse named Lora then called me back. She started asking me routine questions, and then even she was baffled that I still had hair. Now, keep in mind that I had learned how to manipulate my look with headbands and caps. When I took them off at night, I turned into some sort of half-bald creation that was part hillbilly, part monster. It was the worst sight I had ever seen. But during the day, I looked half decent.

"Did you use the cold cap?" Lora asked me.

I responded the same way as before: "No, I just prayed a lot."

Lora thought that was amazing. She, too, was a believer. She had gone through breast cancer a few years back, so we briefly discussed how important we both believed faith had been to getting us through cancer.

Lora explained a little about radiation and how the area that would be radiated might appear red, like it had been sunburned. The radiation treatment would be a quick process but I would need to come in every day, Monday through Friday.

After this brief discussion, Lora asked that I get into a gown and she called the doctor back to speak with me.

I changed into the gown and waited for the doctor to come into the room. I wasn't quite sure what to expect, and I said a little prayer. I simply asked God to not have me need more than a month of radiation. I didn't want to be exposed to too much radiation because, as we all know, it's dangerous.

The doctor knocked and then entered the room, introducing himself. This was déjà vu. Even the doctor looked at me and asked, "Are you wearing a wig or...?"

I felt amazing that everyone was baffled that I didn't have complete hair loss! I responded the same way I had responded the other two times, and then the doctor dove right in, warning me of all the potential short-term and long-term side effects of radiation: difficulty swallowing (because one of the places that would be radiated was my neck area), sharp pain if I bent my neck (seriously?!), damage to my lungs, persistent cough, thyroid issues—oh yeah, and a secondary cancer thanks to radiation. So, you kill one kind of cancer and then another could appear! Isn't that wonderful?

As he listed the potentialities, tears streamed down my face. Hearing those possible side effects was frightening. Then he gave me some good news: I would be exposed to the lowest dose of radiation, and I would need radiation for only three and a half weeks. Once again, God had answered my prayer, and I was grateful for that.

My head was spinning with all of this information, but I was able to digest everything on the drive back to work. I immediately found one of my bosses, Mike, and explained what was going on. We all know how men are very rational and logical, so I was able to vent to Mike about radiation and how I may have issues down the road. "I might have to take thyroid medication for the rest of my life," I nervously explained.

Mike, without hesitation, then responded with the most amazing and logical statement possible: "Taking a thyroid pill every day is better than having fucking cancer." I couldn't help but feel better because what he had said was so true.

I had the rest of the afternoon and evening to digest radiation. Hey, if I could make it through chemo, radiation would be a total cakewalk!

Little did I know, that cake would be poisonous.

June 27, 2016

I returned to the cancer center to have a meeting with both the radiation doctor and radiation technician to prepare for the next step of my journey. Just like on my last visit, I was instructed to get into a gown and wait until I was called. A really cute radiation tech introduced himself to me and took me into the area that the treatment was performed in. He asked me to take my head cap off. I froze. I absolutely did not want him to see what was underneath. Feeling embarrassed, I removed the cute cap I was wearing, exposing the strands of hair that ran wild like a mad scientist.

I was instructed to lie down on the bed that they perform the radiation on. Today, they would be making a mask of my head. I would need to wear this mask every time I had radiation to ensure that I was completely still during the process so no errors would occur. To take things up a notch, I also received a tattoo (like, a legitimate tattoo) of a dot on my lower chest, under my boobs. This dot would be the mark that the radiation laser would hit—again, to ensure that I was getting zapped in the right places.

I lay very still as the tech put what felt like a warm washcloth over my face. It was a wet mesh cloth that would dry in the shape of my head. It was tight and wet and felt weird. Oh, and it gets better: During this process, he needed to take pictures of me, so as I was lying there with my gown basically falling off me, exposing my tiny boobs, with a mesh mask over my entire face, I was having a photo shoot. In that moment, I was tempted to ask the tech for copies of the pictures so I could use them for my online dating profile.

When the mask was dry, it was taken off of me, leaving a mesh pattern imprinted on my face for the next few minutes.

After receiving my new tattoo and mesh head, I was able to leave the cancer center and go to work. I kept thinking, *Gosh, it's not even July yet, and already, I want it to be over with.*

This was my first day of radiation treatment. I was feeling perfectly fine, not nervous or anything. I parked in the VIP parking (in reality, it was a designated space for radiation patients), entered the cancer center (yuck!), and walked straight back to the radiation department. I changed into a cute pink gown that would soon be known as radiation chic, and shortly after, one of the radiation techs called me for my first zap session.

I lay down on the bed, and soon after, the two techs assisted me in putting the mesh mask on my face. It was tight and made me very uncomfortable. Imagine being restrained in something that makes you unable to move your eyes or lips. I tried speaking through the mask. "Wis weels so wange!" I said. (Translation: "This feels so strange!")

I soon became pretty anxious and a tad claustrophobic. One of the techs put oxygen near my nose to help the process. And don't get me started on how I had to lie—I had to keep my hands underneath my butt to ensure that I would keep still during the process. I kept thinking, *Let's please just hurry this along.*

The techs needed to be extremely thorough and precise. This meant that I was in that position for about ten minutes, which honestly felt like ten years. The techs assured me that future sessions would be quicker. They just needed to make sure that I was in the right position today, which is why it took the longest. For the future, it would take less time because they would already have the precise measurements for where I would be radiated.

The radiation itself wasn't painful in any way. I heard a loud buzzing sound, but I didn't feel anything at all. Shortly after the buzzing sound stopped, the techs came and took the mask off my face. Once again, I had a lovely mesh print temporarily tattooed all over my face.

I went back to the changing room to take my gown off and got back into my regular clothes. My dad was in the waiting room. He took me out for breakfast afterward, and I was feeling okay—not wonderful, just okay.

I kept telling myself that I was one day closer to being done with radiation. I was about to be faced with the horrible truth, though: that July was going to be the longest and hardest month of this entire year.

July 7, 2016

Hey, remember that time I thought radiation would be easy? I couldn't have been more wrong. After only three sessions, I wished I could stop. I was plagued with severe nausea and didn't know what to do with myself. At work, I was unable to concentrate. I'd sit at my computer, trying to decide whether I needed to run to the bathroom to throw up. My work was suffering just as much as I was, and I had no idea how I'd continue like this.

I left work on this day before 2 p.m. As I already mentioned, I worked for the best bosses I could ever ask for. Dave and Mike were so understanding and compassionate that it really made the process of cancer treatment much easier.

At home, I tried to lie down and relax. Thankfully, I didn't throw up. I stayed in bed, watching trashy reality TV to get my mind off how I felt. I went to bed early, hoping my night would go super-slow. I was absolutely in no rush to go back for another radiation session the next day.

July 8, 2016

I managed to get through work until about 3:30 today, when Dave decided to close the office down and let us all go home early. *Thank you, God!* I screamed in my head. It was another day of feeling nauseous from the radiation, and I still had no idea why it was happening.

When I got home from work, my dad called to check up on me. I told him how nauseous I had been in the past two days, and he innocently asked, "Why don't you take those nausea pills that you took when you were going for chemo?"

I quickly replied, "Dad, I need to call you back." Then I ran to the bathroom and got sick, thinking, *You've got to be kidding me. I thought this was behind me.*

Unfortunately, I was still at a very sensitive point, where anything relating to chemo could set me off. Certain smells could make me cry instantaneously—for example, the smell of the laundry detergent that my mom used. When I was staying with my parents as I recovered from each round of chemo, my mom would wash my clothes with a specific laundry detergent. After that, if I caught a whiff of that smell, I would begin to cry immediately as I was taken back to those horrible memories.

No, I'm not making this up. I was beyond sensitive, and anything could set me off at any time, so when my dad mentioned those pills, it brought back traumatic memories of chemo. Even putting those pills in my mouth after chemo would make me dry-heave immediately.

I spent the rest of my night exactly as I had the previous night: in bed, watching trashy reality shows to get my mind off how sick I felt. I forgot about my current situation as I watched the people on TV live glamorous, unrealistic lives in their huge homes and fancy cars.

I was miserable and didn't know what do with myself, so I kept telling myself that July would be over soon. Soon, I would be healthy again. Soon, I would feel normal again.

"Soon" felt so far away, but I knew I needed to keep fighting.

July 11, 2016

"Why is this happening?" I asked one of the radiation techs before my next radiation session began. "Is nausea normal during radiation?"

The tech looked at me, puzzled at what I was going through, and replied, "No, it's not. If we were radiating your stomach, then yes, it would be normal. We aren't anywhere close to your stomach, though."

I was frustrated that I didn't have an answer for why I was feeling so sick from radiation. Even the radiation doctor himself was confused, so I knew I needed to try to deal with it as best I could.

There was no possible way I could have gone to work after this day's treatment. As soon as I got home from my radiation session, I went straight to bed and didn't move. Then my sister called me, telling me she had something for me and was coming over.

She walked in holding a bag. I couldn't believe I hadn't tried this sooner, even during chemo. The bag contained edibles, as in edible marijuana products. She had bought an assortment of edible gummy candies, brownies, and chocolate for me. (Remember that I live in Colorado, and it is legal here to simply go to a dispensary and purchase pot if you are 21 or older.)

"God bless you," I told her. My sister had gone to the dispensary and explained my situation to one of the employees, and he had recommended these products to help with my nausea. I immediately ate one gummy candy and waited for it to take effect. Sure enough, it worked like a charm.

I know what you might be thinking: How could you be a Christian and eat edibles? I'm sure we could debate this all day, but here is what I believe: Marijuana is legal in Colorado and is all-natural. People have been using marijuana for years to help with their illness and even cure it. I have read a handful of articles about cannabis oil curing cancer. Yes, *curing* it. Marijuana, in my opinion, is a better alternative to the medications we get from the drugstore. A lot of those medications have side effects that can hurt us down the road. When it comes to people who are fighting cancer, I 100 percent support the use of medicinal marijuana, especially if they have nausea like I did. I would get sick just *thinking* of my normal medication! I felt that at this point, my only option was to resort to medicinal marijuana, and I was completely fine with that. I see nothing wrong with it.

Now, for those of you who do not live in a state where marijuana is legal, I strongly advise that you obtain a medical marijuana card if it is available in your state so you have access to marijuana the legal way. I don't condone anything being done illegally.

With that said, I started to feel much better whenever I would eat an edible. And I was able to sleep like a baby. It was magical.

July 15, 2016

The past ten days had felt like one big bout of déjà vu. Everything became routine and structured, and there was no escaping it. Every morning, I would pull into the cancer center's parking lot at approximately 7:30 a.m. I would park in the VIP section and take a moment to calm my nerves before walking in. Next, I would cover my nose with a handkerchief as soon as I entered the cancer center because if I smelled *that smell*, I would totally lose it. I would speed-walk from the entrance of the cancer center to the radiation department in the back. Then I would put my belongings in a locker and change into a pink, radiation chic gown and wait for one of the radiation techs to call my name. And then it was time for the zapping.

After the session was over, I would change back into my clothes and once again speed-walk from the radiation department to the exit, holding my breath, relying on my handkerchief to protect my nose from any unwanted odors, run out through the vestibule, and take a deep breath of fresh air. Each and every time I exited the cancer center, I felt like an inmate who had just been released from prison. I tried to overdose on fresh air as I walked to my car. In my car, I would tell myself, "I did it! One day closer to being done!"

Some people accomplish things like graduating from nursing school, raising a child, or winning a prestigious award. In those moments, my greatest accomplishment was getting out of the cancer center without throwing up. Baby steps... baby steps.

July 17, 2016

So, this is where things start to go from bad to worse. I was having dinner with my dad and sister. My dad had cooked us penne with vodka sauce. It had some spices in it, but nothing too crazy. We began eating, but three bites in, I thought I was going to die. Suddenly, my entire chest started burning. I could barely breathe. I stood up from the table and ran outside to get some fresh air. I started having a coughing spell. *What the hell is happening to me?* I kept asking myself.

My dad and sister followed me outside, and in between coughing and gasping for air, I explained how I was feeling. My sister went inside to get me a glass of milk with the hope that it would coat my chest and help ease the burning sensation. It helped a little bit.

I stood outside for a little while longer, and the burning sensation became a bit more tolerable. This sensation was different from the pains I had felt when I would drink alcohol prior to being diagnosed, and I knew it was different than those pains connected to Hodgkin's.

Then I remembered that one of the side effects of radiation was esophagitis, or an inflamed esophagus. My doctor had warned me about this, but he hadn't told me how intense it was going to be.

Shortly after, I ended up getting sick and throwing up my guts. Let me tell you something: Throwing up in itself is the worst thing ever. Throwing up when your esophagus burns? There aren't any words to describe that.

Later that night, I came to the sad realization that this horrible feeling of my esophagus being inflamed wasn't going away anytime soon. On top of that, I began experiencing difficulty swallowing, another side effect of radiation. As much as I wanted to feel sorry for myself, though, I couldn't, because I knew this was only temporary. I had to continue to fight and be strong. I knew I was close to being done with this forever.

July 18, 2016

"Was it the vodka sauce that did me in?" I eagerly asked one of the techs. She said it had nothing to do with that. She explained that the feeling I had experienced the night before was common for radiation patients. All at once, it can hit you hard. What I had experienced was completely normal.

As if eating wasn't hard enough because I couldn't stomach so many foods, it had now gotten harder. For obvious reasons, the techs told me to avoid spicy and sour foods while I was plagued with esophagitis. They also recommended I take some liquid antacid prior to eating to coat my esophagus and stomach.

After radiation was over, I went back to my car to head to work. Before turning my car on, I looked over at my passenger side. There sat Sonia, waiting for me to put her on. I no longer had a choice. I was getting tired of wearing head caps, which basically screamed that I was a cancer patient, so I put Sonia on and wore her to work for the very first time. I was beyond insecure.

I was pretty certain that everyone in the office knew of my situation by now. I mean, it had become blatantly obvious. I was missing tons of work, was penciling in my eyebrows, and had less hair every single day. The head caps were also a dead giveaway, so it now felt like a giant elephant in the room: the cancer elephant. Still, though, I didn't make an official announcement. I guess Sonia was the unofficial announcement.

I was feeling all sorts of nervous wearing her, and I felt super self-conscious. I had decided that if someone were to ask about my wig, I would make a light joke such as "Yeah, today is Bring Your Wig to Work Day. Did you not get the memo?"

Luckily, because everyone I work with is so nice, all I received were compliments. No one pried or asked questions; they simply said things like "You look adorable" and "I love it!"

Once I had gotten that over with, I started to feel less insecure and more relaxed.

For lunch that afternoon, I ate a small piece of chicken, roasted asparagus, and mushrooms. As delicious as this meal was, I couldn't finish even half of it. Not only was swallowing a difficult process, but once the food went down, it burned. I became more miserable with every bite.

Another major issue I was dealing with was dehydration. Just like during chemo, I had no desire to drink water. During chemo, water had sometimes tasted metallic; this time around, it didn't taste metallic, just weird, and I couldn't bring myself to drink.

I started to drink all-natural flavored carbonated water because I was able to get that down without gagging. Regular water, though, wasn't an option. It truly was a struggle, and I knew how dehydrated I was. There was nothing I could do about it, though. I was doing the best I could, but when you are sick and feel like crap, suddenly, part of you can't care less about drinking fluids like you are supposed to. At this point, the only thing I was hoping for was to stop feeling so damn sick. Nausea, esophagitis, difficulty swallowing, and dehydration—I was one hot mess.

July 22, 2016

It finally happened. Although the typical cancer patient goes through it, I had been certain that it wouldn't happen to me. But it did.

I finally faced reality and said good-bye to all of my hair. Although I had been done with chemo for well over a month, the poison was still in my system. My hair was still thinning, with no intention of stopping. At this point, I was wearing Sonia to work daily. I could no longer wear headbands because they couldn't cover up the large bald patches in the back of my head. I was almost entirely bald. The part of my head that wasn't bald had only a few strands of hair on either side of my head. I looked ridiculous. It had finally come to the point that I needed to cut off those strands.

I was alone in my apartment. I stepped into my bathroom nervously. Although I wasn't doing anything extreme like shaving my head, it was still an emotional and nerve-wracking moment. It wasn't just that I was cutting my hair, but that I hadn't thought this would happen. (Although let's be real, I never thought I would have cancer, either!) Suddenly, things became even more real to me, if that makes sense. This was the moment that would, in my opinion, solidify me being a cancer patient. Up until this point, I had been able to flaunt my strands of hair and be proud that I had not gone bald. Well, not anymore.

I used a pair of scissors to begin cutting the straggly strands of hair on my head. Snip, snip, snip. In less than one minute, it was over. I cried for less than five minutes, but after that, I never cried over my hair again.

I will be completely honest with you. The bald look wasn't nearly as terrifying as I had imagined it would be. Yeah, you look different and feel really strange, but after I had spent fewer than five minutes crying, my bald head never bothered me again. In fact, I began flaunting it to my closest friends. I'd send them pictures of me with funny captions.

I knew I wasn't going to be bald forever, and I knew my bald head was my "badge of honor," as my aunt Janis called it. It was a symbol that the chemo worked and I had survived cancer. I was unashamed of what I looked like, and I knew that I was still beautiful. In fact, this was probably the most beautiful I have ever looked.

July 25, 2016

The nausea and vomiting were still occurring—relentlessly. For the past two mornings, as soon as I had woken up, I had thrown up. I was down to 109 pounds, which meant I had lost five pounds in one week. I didn't let this get the best of me, though; I did my very best to keep a good attitude despite feeling so terrible. I began joking with my friends that I was going to invent a new diet plan that would make me millions. "It's called the radiation diet," I joked. "It's guaranteed to get you down to your birth weight in less than a month. All you need to do is go for radiation. You can barely eat, and you throw up all the time. It's proven to work, and there's a money-back guarantee."

At my radiation session on this morning, I expressed my concern about my vomiting to the doctor. I was extremely nervous about possibly needing to throw up as I was confined in that mask for treatment. I could die! The doctor agreed with me and told me to skip radiation that day and come back tomorrow. This meant that July 29—not July 28—would be my last day. You better believe that this day was marked on my calendar with multiple exclamation points!

I was so sick that my mom had to drive me to the cancer center that morning. I couldn't go to work, so I decided to spend the morning at my parents' house with them, because I didn't want to be alone.

On the drive home, my mom needed to pull over so I could throw up. "The radiation diet is working!" I joked. "Just a few more pounds and I'll be down to my birth weight."

I spent the rest of the day trying to relax and, more importantly, trying to drink. I kept a big bottle of alkaline water with me the whole day and did my best to take sips every few minutes. It was harder than it sounds, but I managed to do the best I could.

I kept focusing on the fact that I was almost done with radiation. I was absolutely thrilled. I was one step closer to getting back to being my old self again. Whenever life started to seem really difficult, I went back to my mental happy place. I would simply focus on my goals for when I got better, and how happy I was going to be. I was also going to be moving to a new, beautiful apartment on August 20, so that gave me something to really look forward to.

My dad also kept reminding me of Psalm 23:4: "Even though I walk through the valley of the shadow of death, I will fear no evil, for you are with me; your rod and your staff, they comfort me." My dad explained, "Notice how it says, 'I *walk through* the valley,' instead of 'I'm staying in the valley'? It's because this is temporary. You are walking through the valley, but you are not there permanently." His words were true, and I was encouraged by them.

This cancer is not permanent, and you need to tell yourself that every day. This is temporary. Never forget that.

July 29, 2016

This was it! I was so excited that I wanted to shout with joy. This was my last day of déjà vu. My last day of my routine of darting through the cancer center with my trusty handkerchief. My last day of wearing the radiation chic gown. My last day of being confined in that horrible mask. My last day of cancer treatment.

When the zap session was over, all of the techs gave me hugs. Before I left, I met with Lora because she had some follow-up questions for me, and I made sure that she knew how much I appreciated her and all the staff. I felt blessed to have had such wonderful people to help me during such a bad time. I gave Lora a giant hug and then left the cancer center excitedly, screaming, *I did it!* in my head.

As I drove out of the cancer center's parking lot, I boldly declared that I would *never* be diagnosed with a disease ever again. This was it, I declared. This was finally it.

August 2, 2016

The past few days had been rough. On Saturday and Sunday mornings, I had thrown up as soon as I had woken up. Then, Monday and this day, my mornings were filled with dry heaves. I was still extremely dehydrated and, overall, a hot mess.

My follow-up appointment with Dr. J was today, at a different location—the cancer center's location in midtown Denver, where I had originally met Dr. J on February 9, when I was diagnosed. I had made my appointment at this location because the other location, where I had received treatment for so long, made me feel so sick that I couldn't deal with it. So there I was at the other location, which held no chemo memories, no radiation memories, and no putrid smell. It was just a normal, average building, in my opinion.

I had always enjoyed seeing Dr. J. Since Day 1, I had felt positive and genuine vibes from him, and I was beyond blessed having him as my oncologist.

The appointment was pretty straightforward: The nurses checked my vitals, and then Dr. J asked if I had any concerns or questions. That's when I asked him the most important question: "So, when am I able to officially be declared cancer-free?"

That's when he said, "It's safe to say you are now cured of your disease."

My heart danced with joy. What beautiful words! He used the word "cured"! The words "cured" and "cancer" together were music to my ears, like a song sung by angels. I was on cloud nine. I was so beyond thrilled, there simply were no words to describe it.

Dr. J shook my hand and told me to make an appointment to come see him in October for a follow-up. The plan was for me to see him in October, have another PET scan in December, and then finally, finally get the awful, hideous port taken out after my PET scan came back normal.

I was finally on the mend. It was all going to be better from this point on. *Thank you, God,* I kept repeating.

August 3, 2016

This was the first day I had felt better since beginning radiation. As I walked outside to my car to leave for work, I took a moment to look around me. An abundance of sunshine was beaming down on me. In that moment, I felt almost completely back to normal. No nausea, no dry heaves, no getting sick. I felt fine. I knew deep down that from this point on, I would start feeling better by the day. It was time for me to get my life back.

Today, I got to celebrate my 29th birthday. This birthday was epic because I got to celebrate this new year of life as a cancer survivor. I was able to drink wine and not have the horrible pains in my chest and arms that were connected to Hodgkin's. I was able to eat food again without esophagitis or difficulty swallowing. I got to kick off this next year of my life as a person who had conquered cancer and proved that faith and prayer are more powerful than anything else in the world. This was the most special birthday I had ever had. I felt blessed, renewed, and on top of the world.

I conquered cancer. I laughed in the storm even when life got difficult. I did it. I did it! I did it because of God's goodness. All of the credit goes to Him. I have been healed because I knew deep down in my heart that no weapon formed against me would ever prosper, and because what was meant for my harm, God was now going to use for my good. It was as simple as that.

Final Thoughts

So, is this where my story ends? No. This is where my story is just beginning. This journey was simply a chapter in my life. I am about to turn the page to a brand new chapter. The next chapter is filled with an abundance of health, happiness, and blessings. I have waited so long to turn the page and get to the next chapter. Now, it's finally happening.

I want you to know that you are going to be in your next chapter sooner than you think. I wholeheartedly believe that if you have the right attitude and a whole lot of faith, nothing can stop you. You simply need to believe that God can heal you. He healed me of Hodgkin's lymphoma, He healed my sister of melanoma, and He has healed numerous others of all different types of cancer, so you need to believe that He will heal you also. Wake up every day and thank God that you are one step closer to being declared cancer-free. God is moved by our faith, not by our complaining. Start believing that God is in control.

The truth is, we are all going to be faced with situations in life that feel unfair. Situations that make us feel uncomfortable. Situations that don't make sense. The key to getting through these difficult times, in my opinion, is putting all of your trust in God. You need to realize that He is in control and that all things are going to work together for your good. It's okay if something doesn't make sense to you; it makes sense to God, and that's all that matters. Our job is to have enough faith to believe that we *will* get better, that we *will* be healed of cancer and we *will* get through these difficult times. My sister and I are proof that this really works. She and I both stayed strong, and now we are completely healed.

Keep fighting, and never, never give up. God's got your back, always.

CPSIA information can be obtained
at www.ICGtesting.com
Printed in the USA
FSOW01n0747130817
37549FS

9 781457 556401